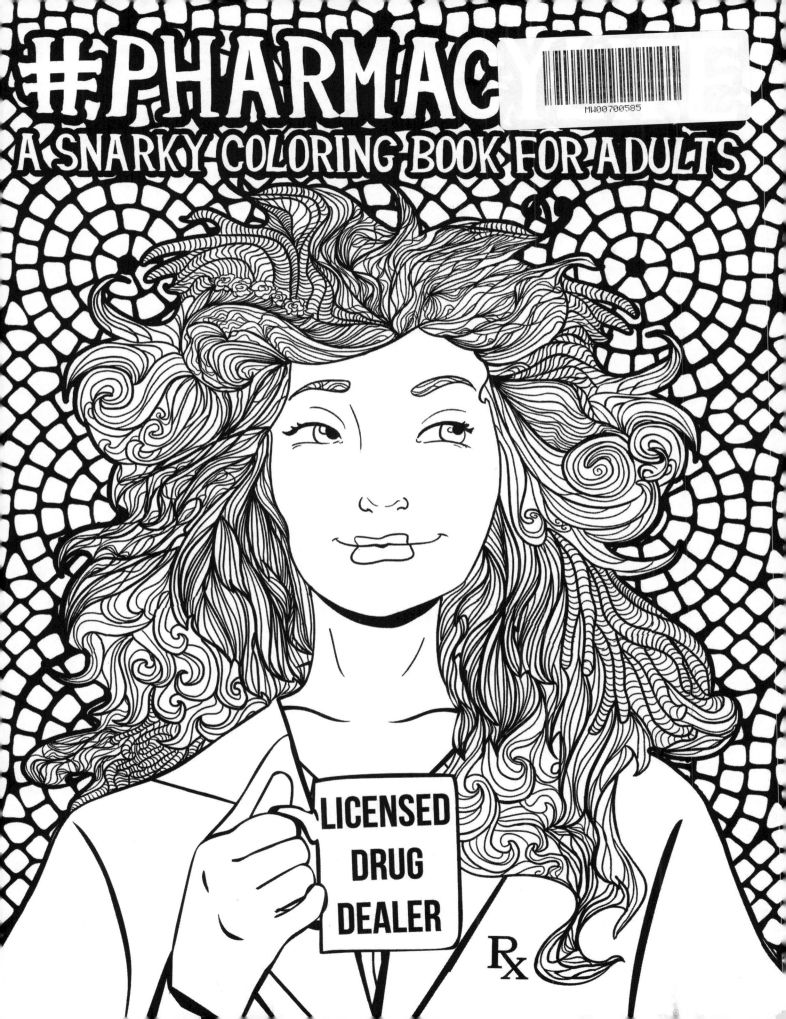

#PHARMACY
A SNARKY COLORING BOOK FOR ADULTS

LICENSED DRUG DEALER

Rx

Want free goodies?
Email us at freebies@pbleu.com

@papeteriebleu

Papeterie Bleu

Shop our other books at
www.pbleu.com

Wholesale distribution through Ingram Content Group
www.ingramcontent.com/publishers/distribution/wholesale

For questions and customer service, email us at
support@pbleu.com

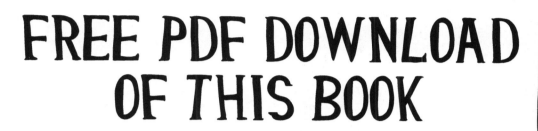
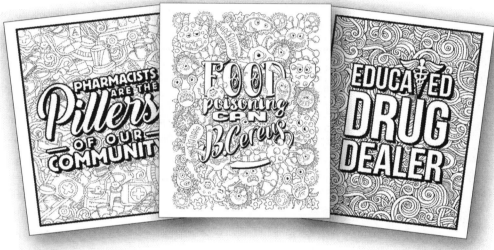
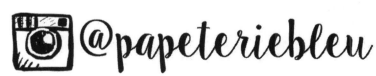
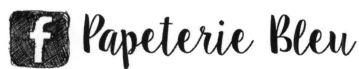

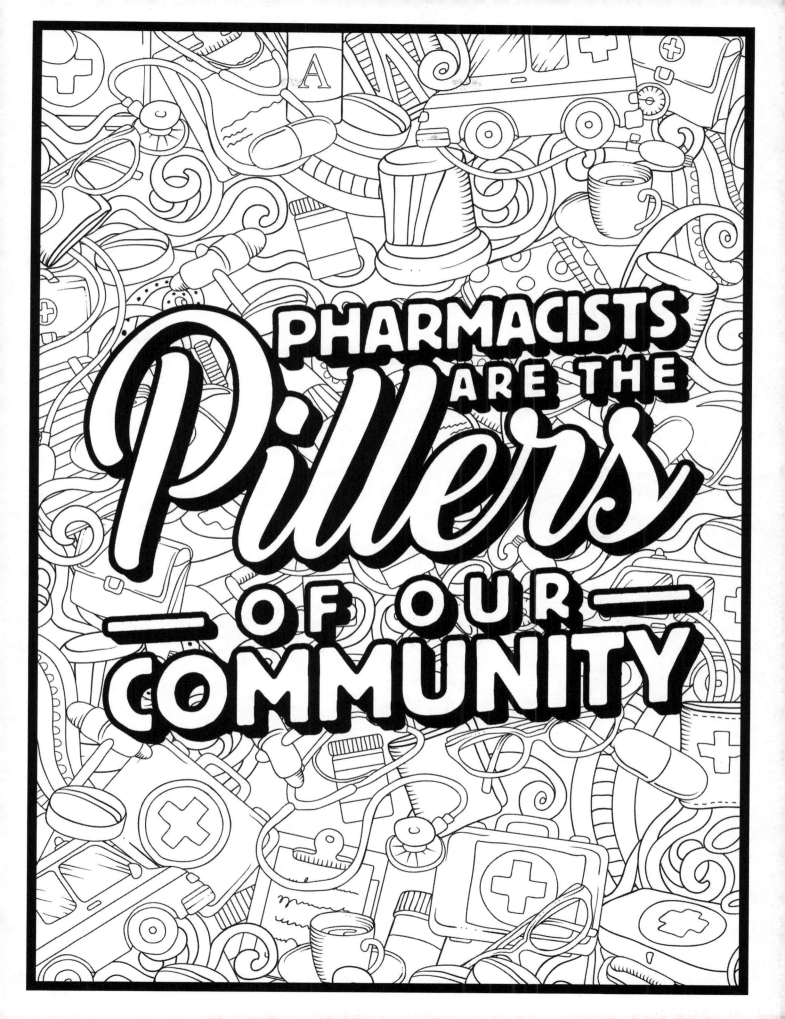

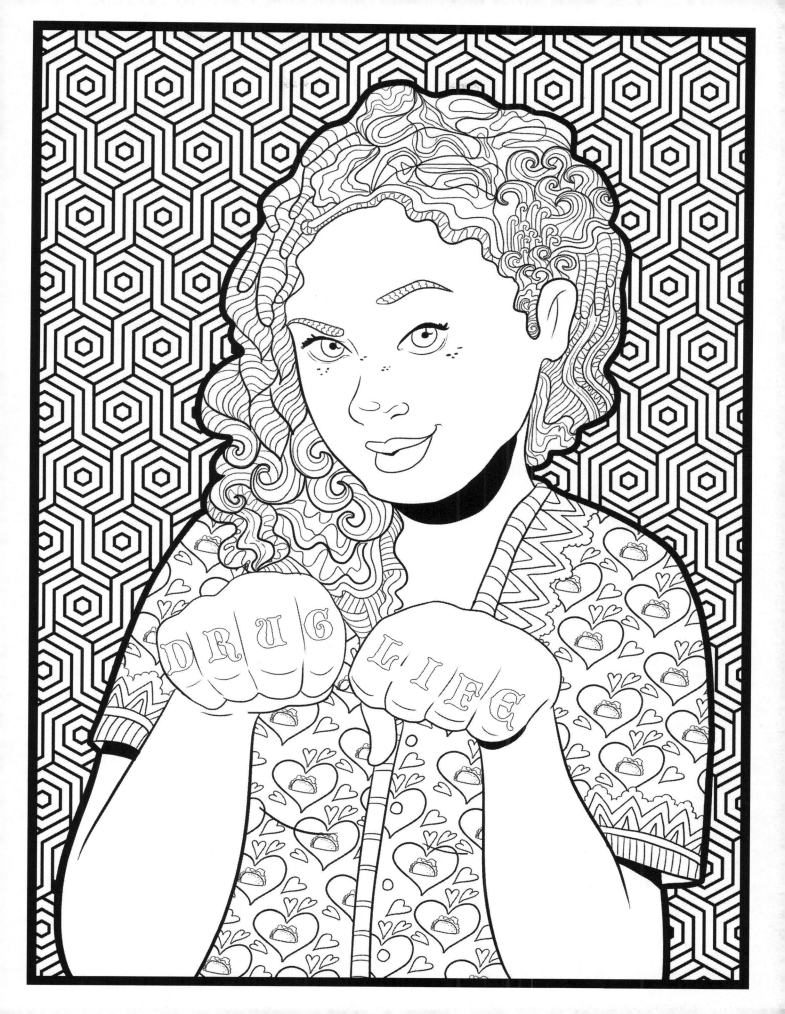

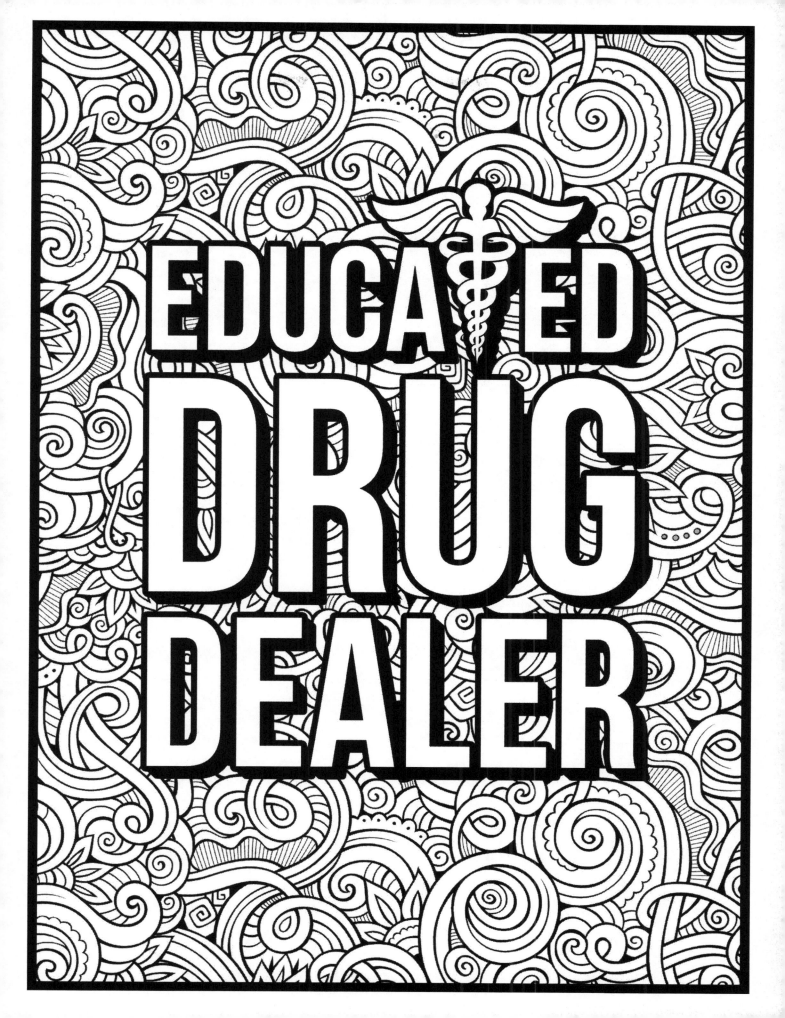

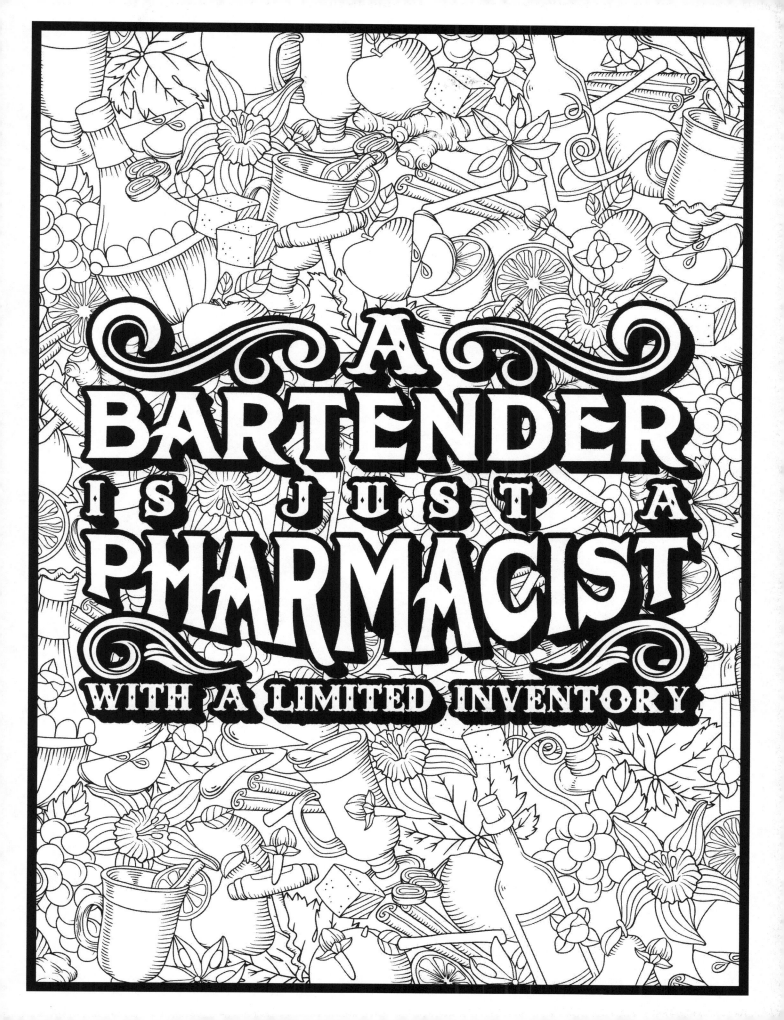

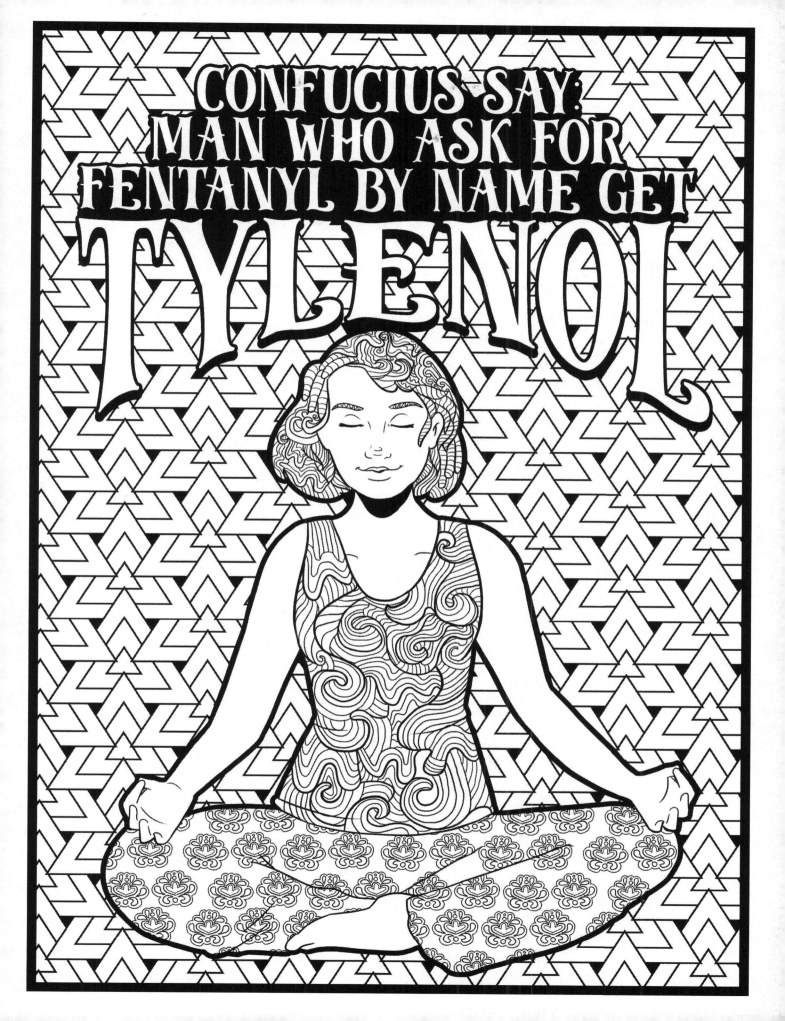

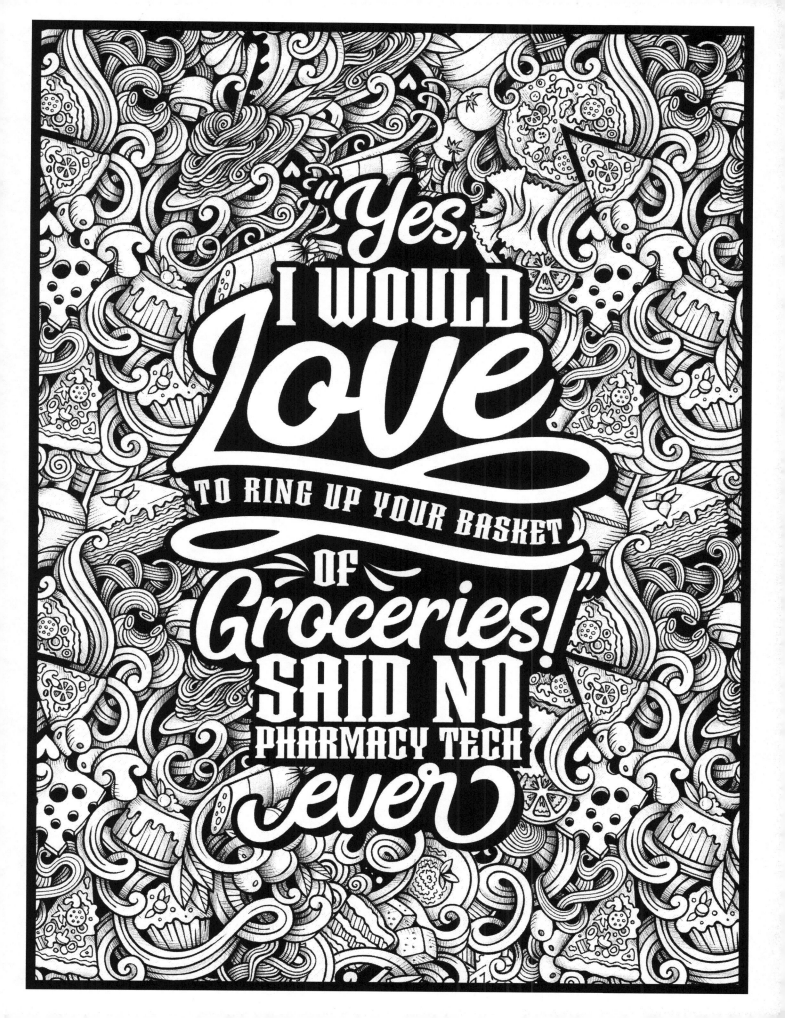

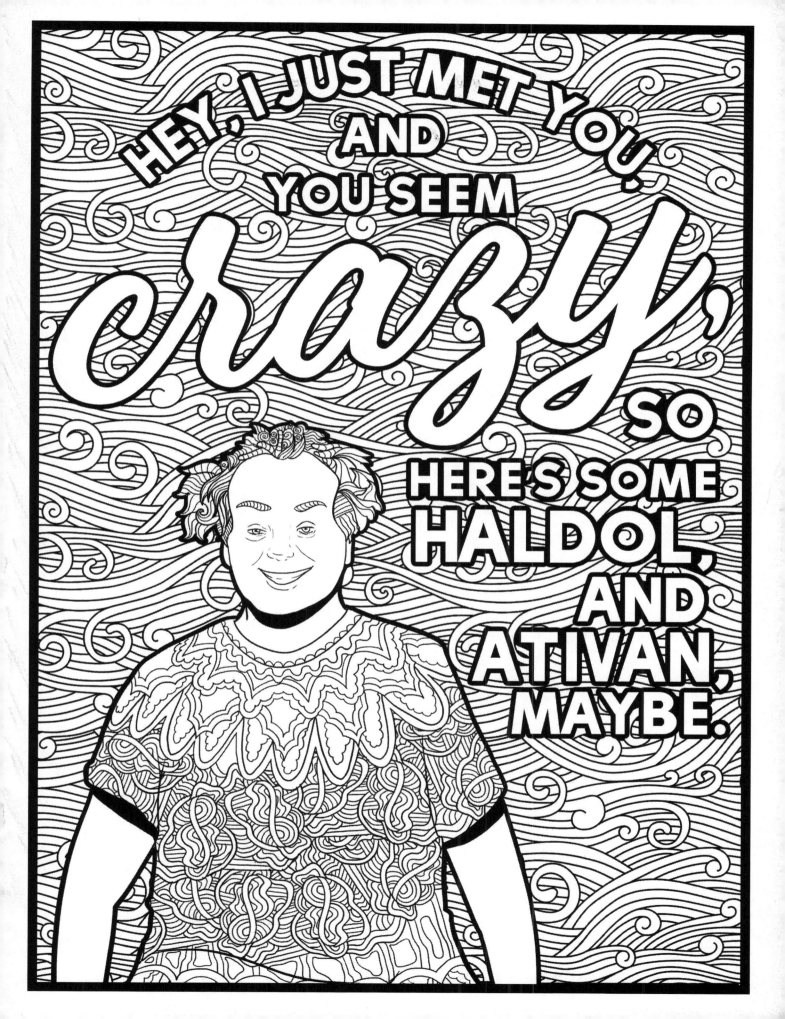

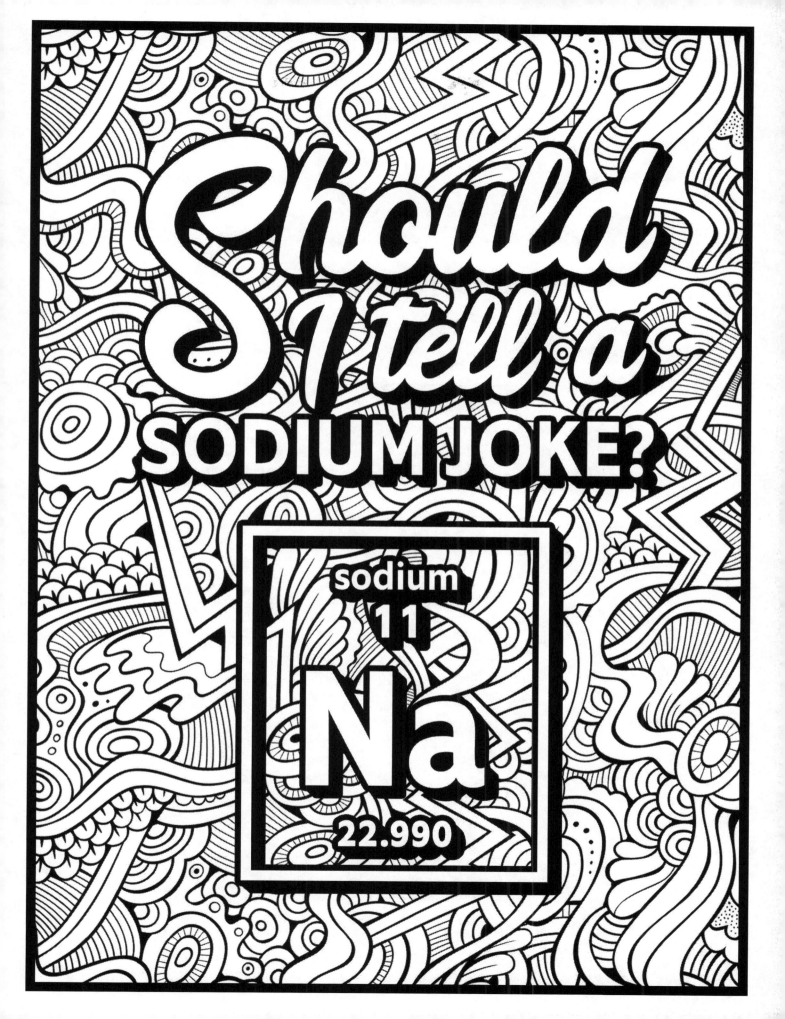

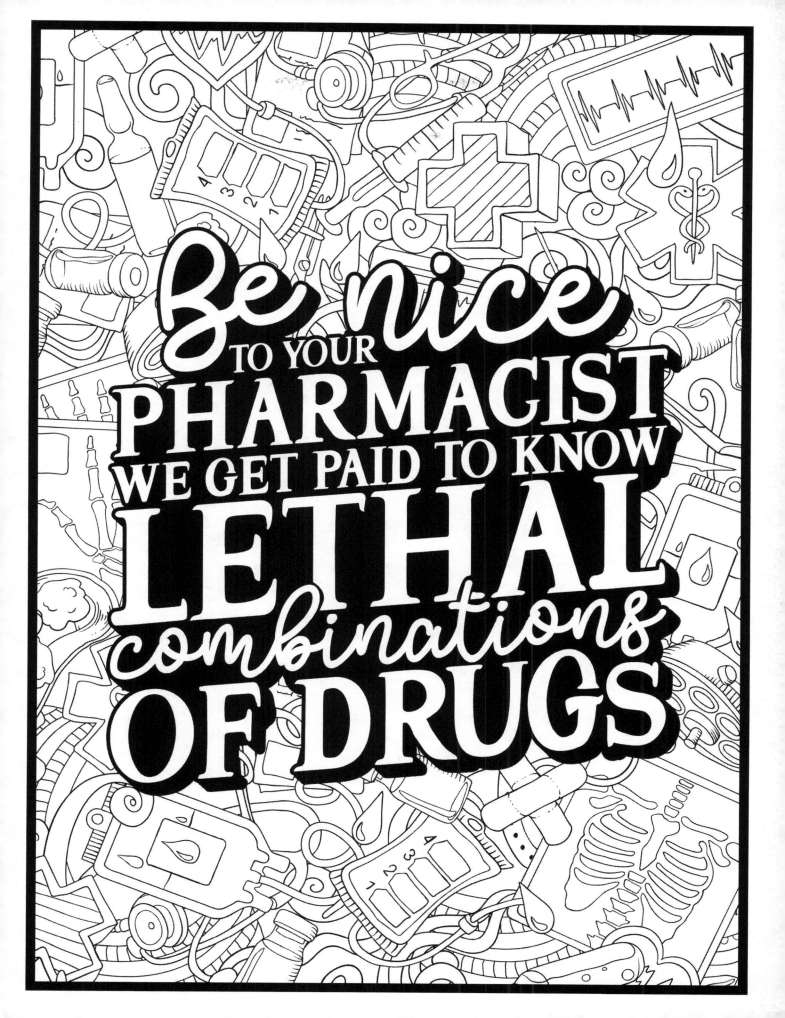

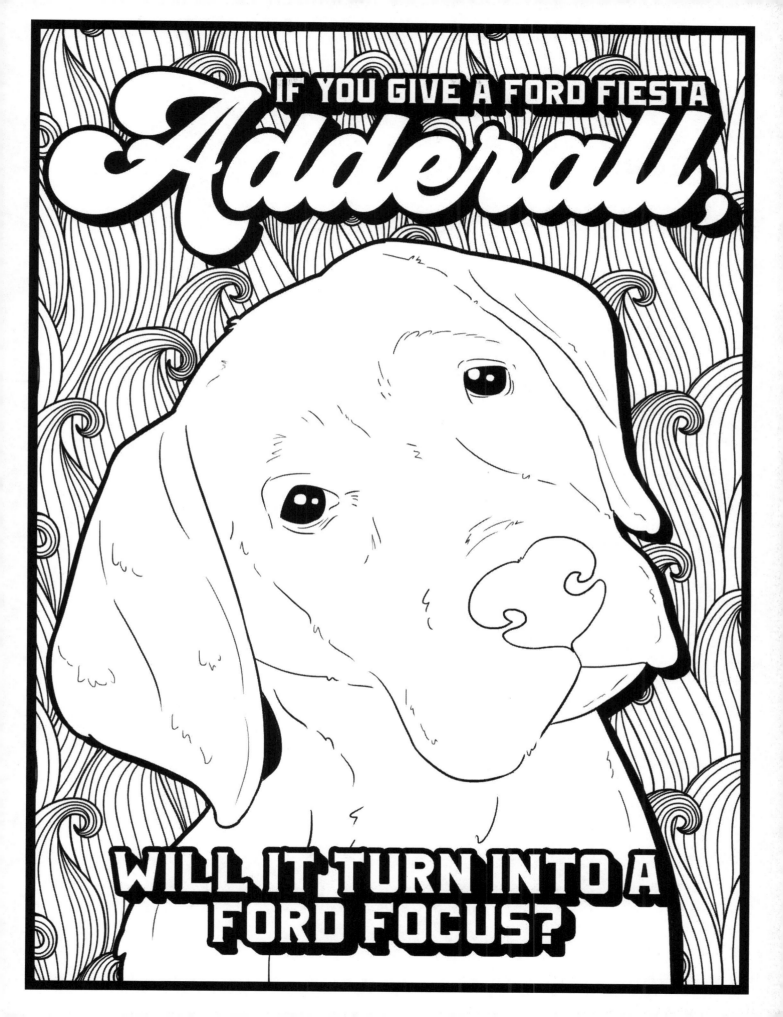

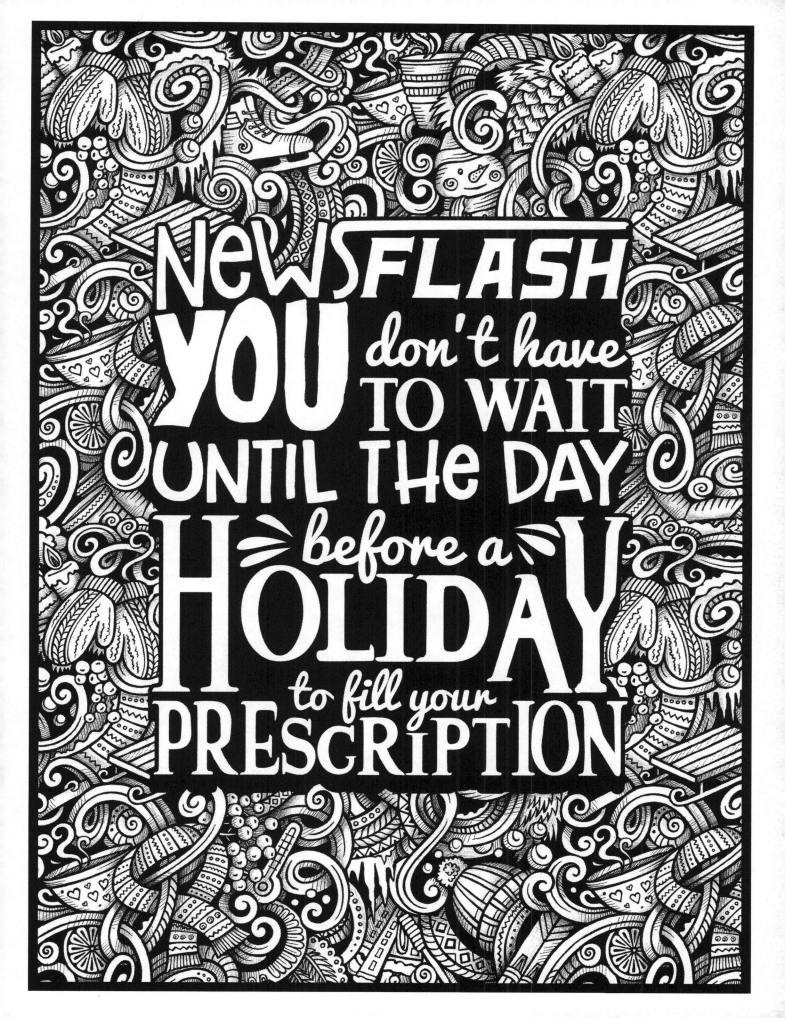

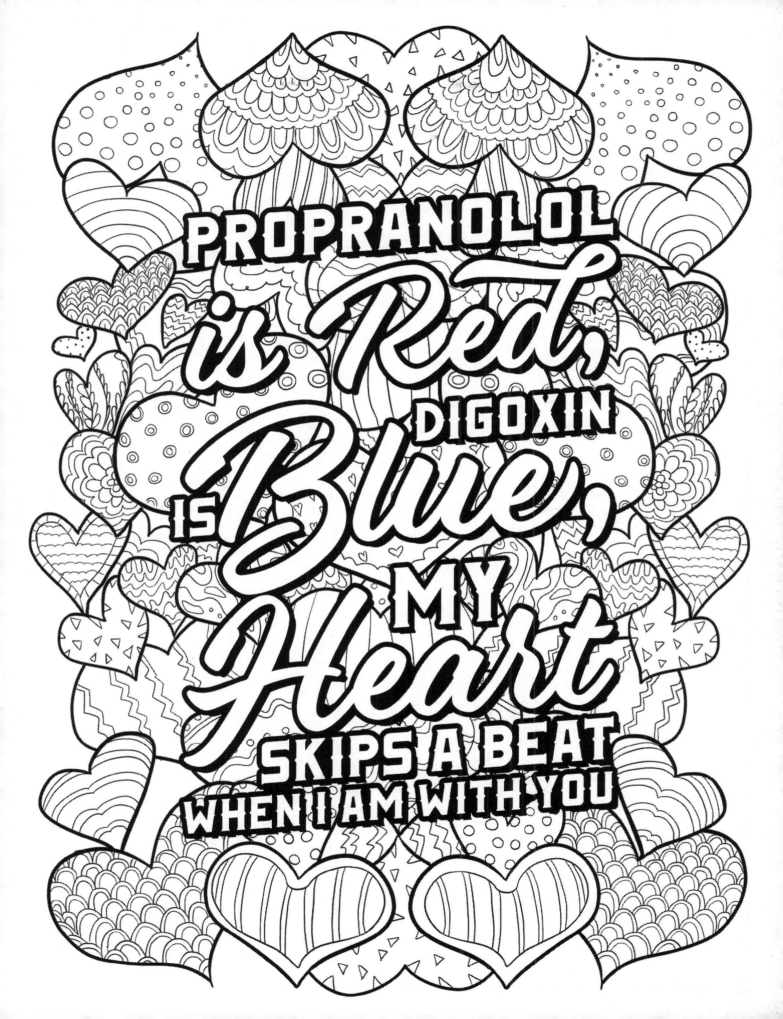

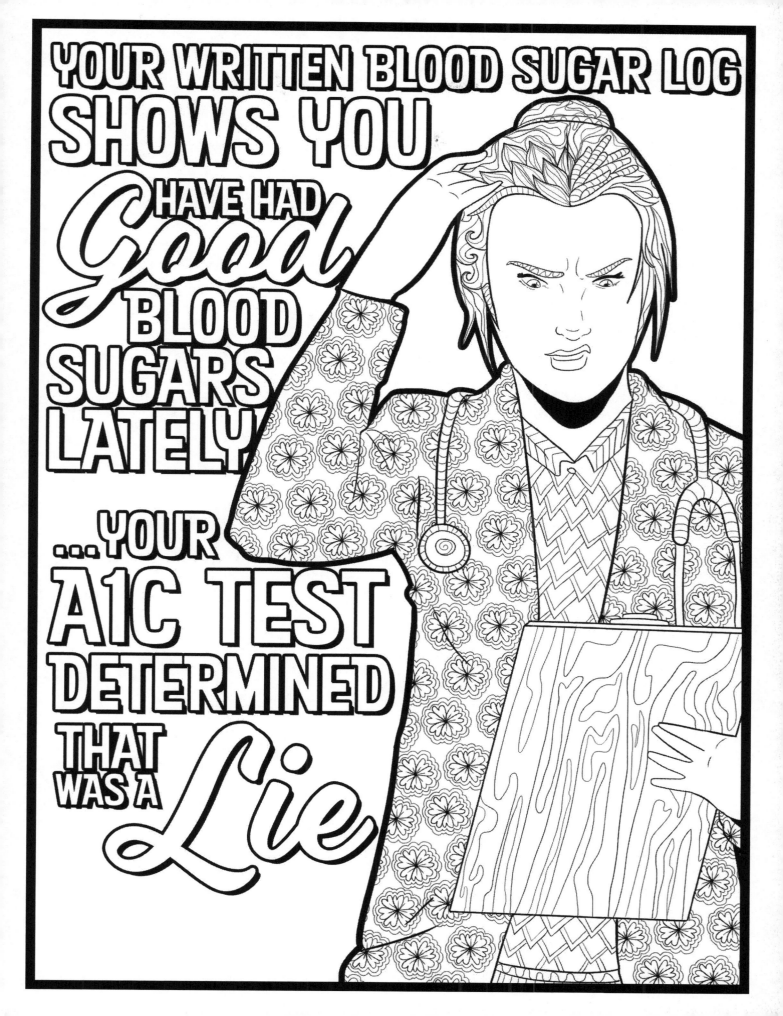

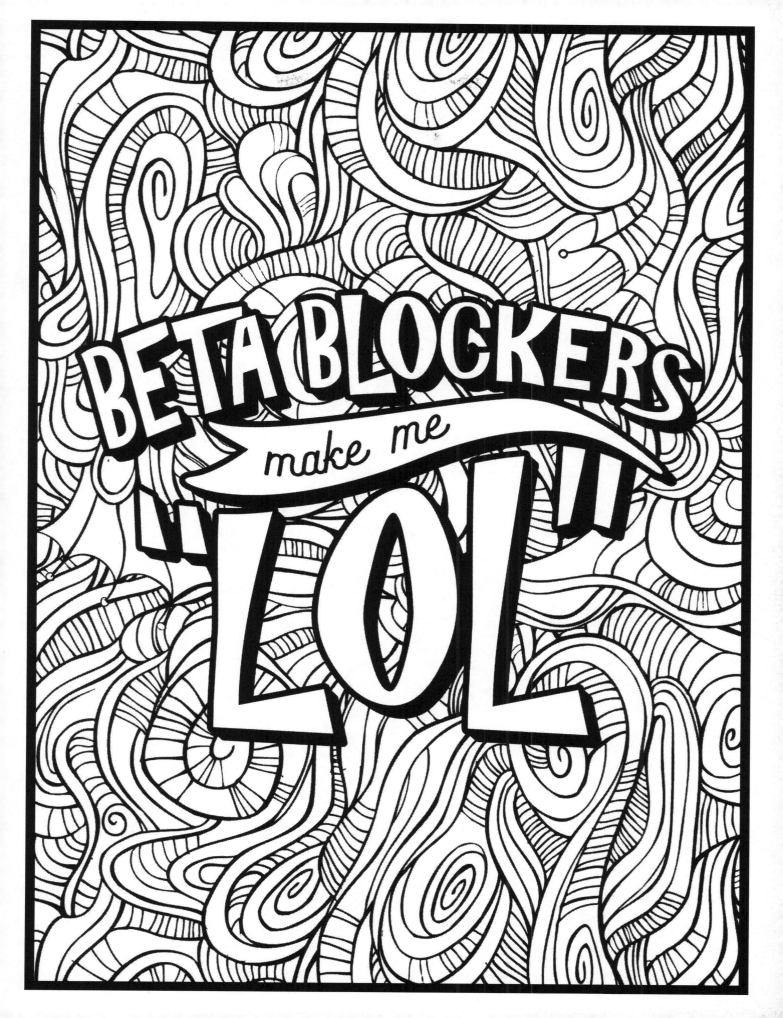

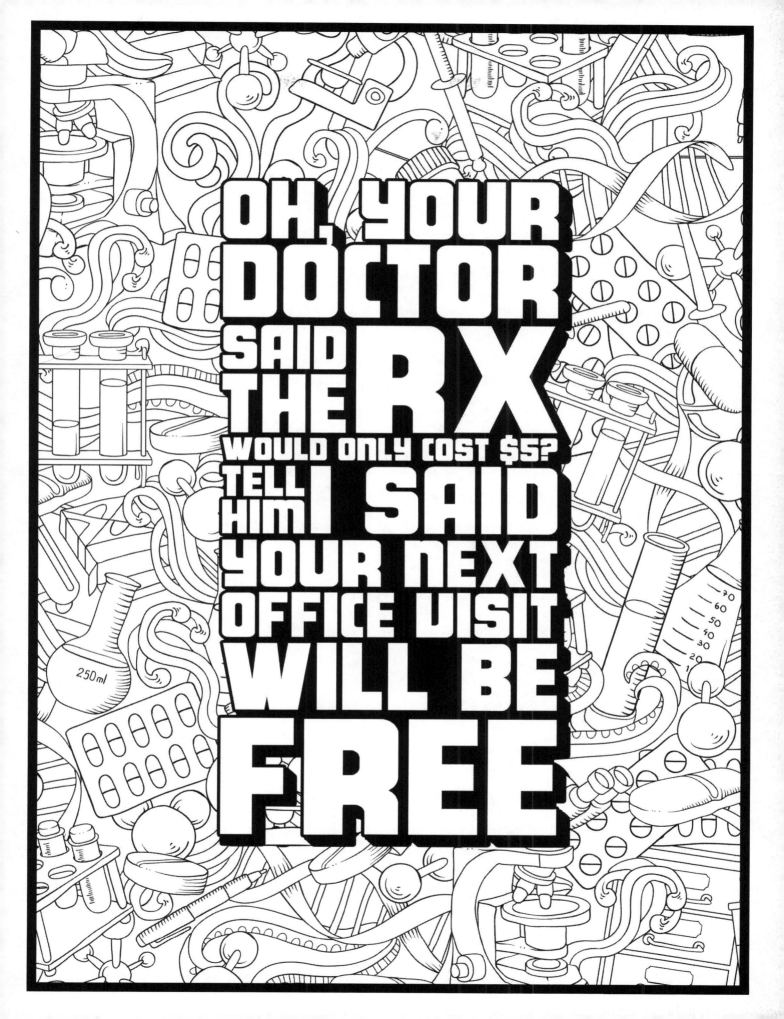

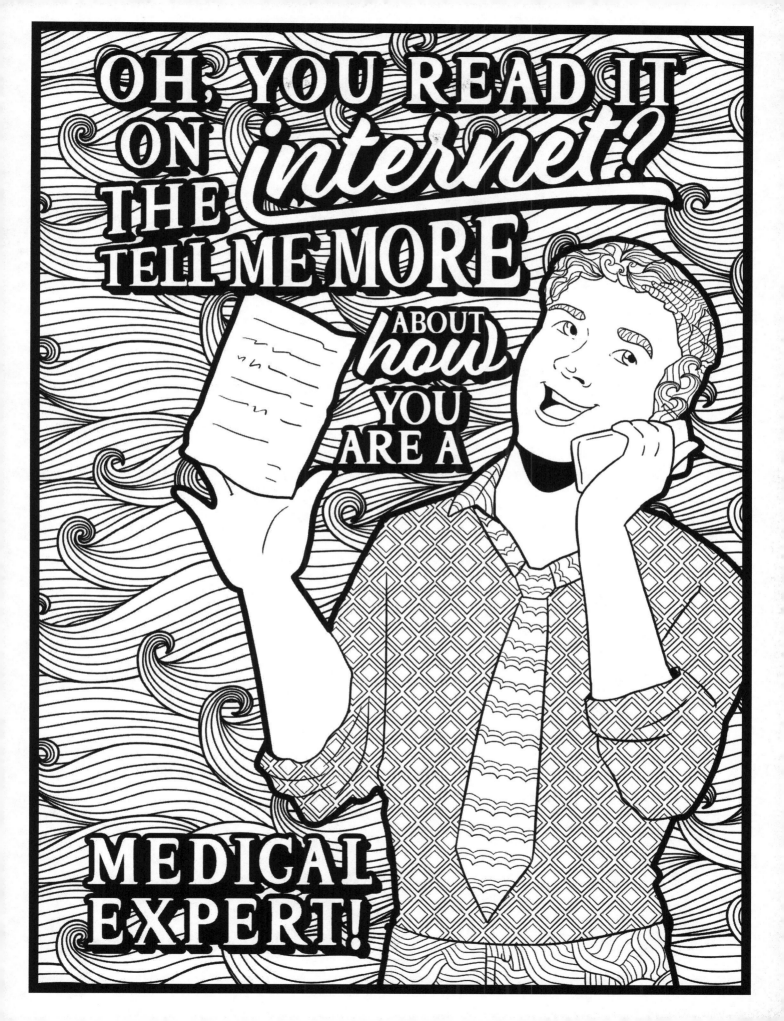

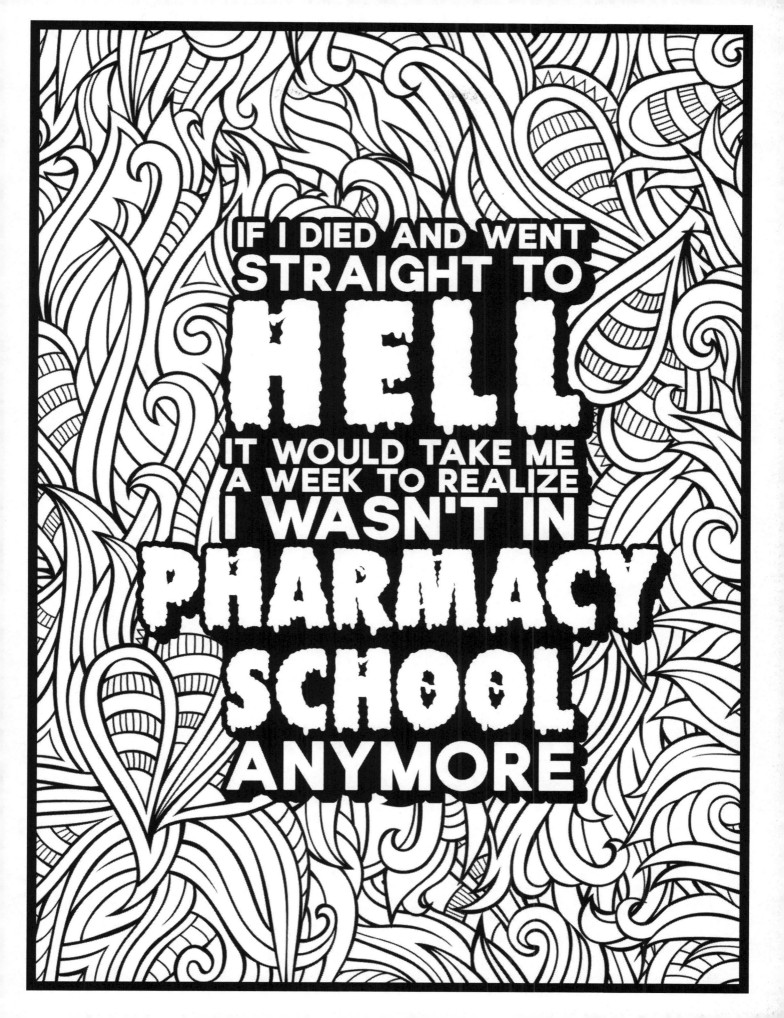

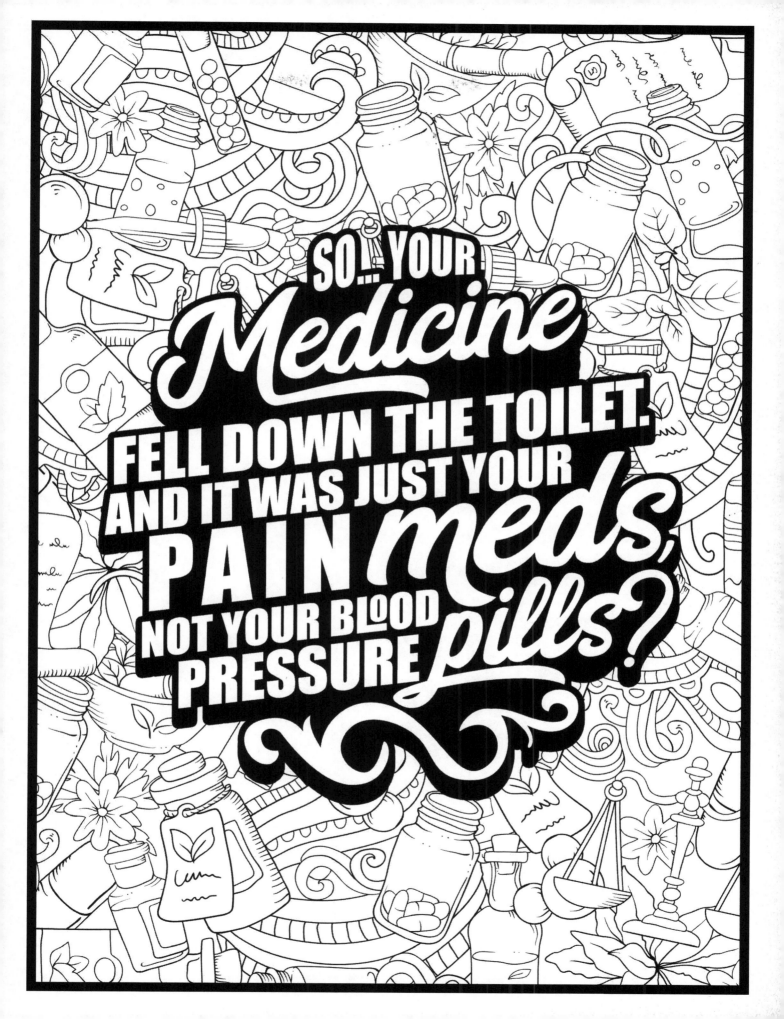

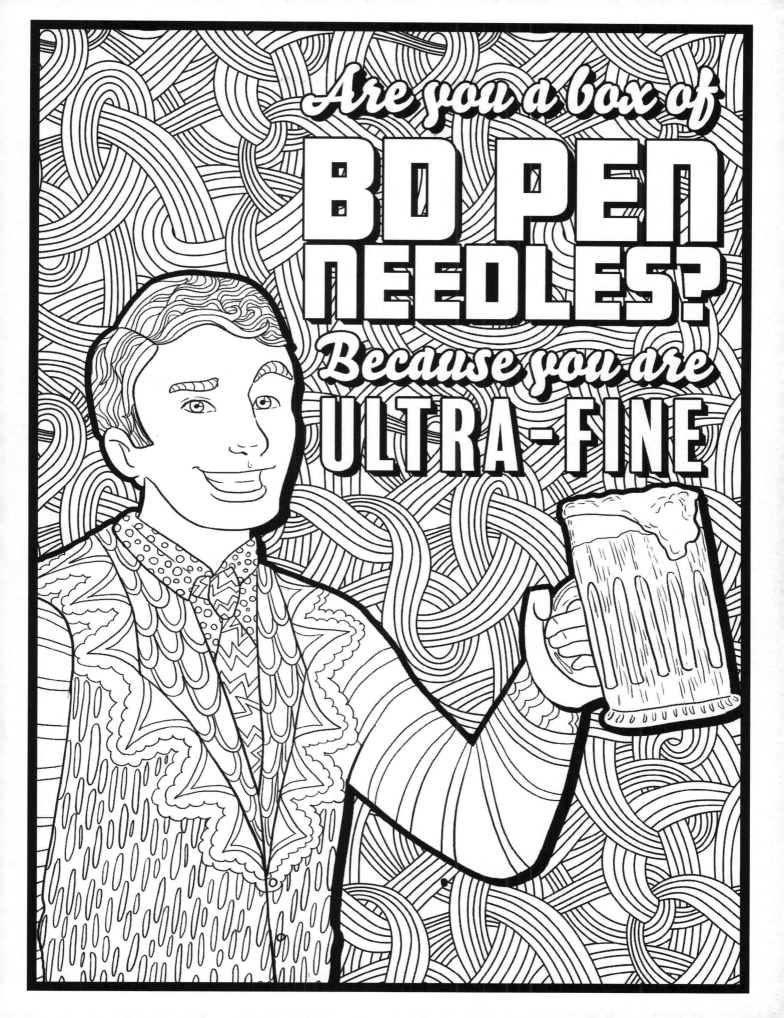

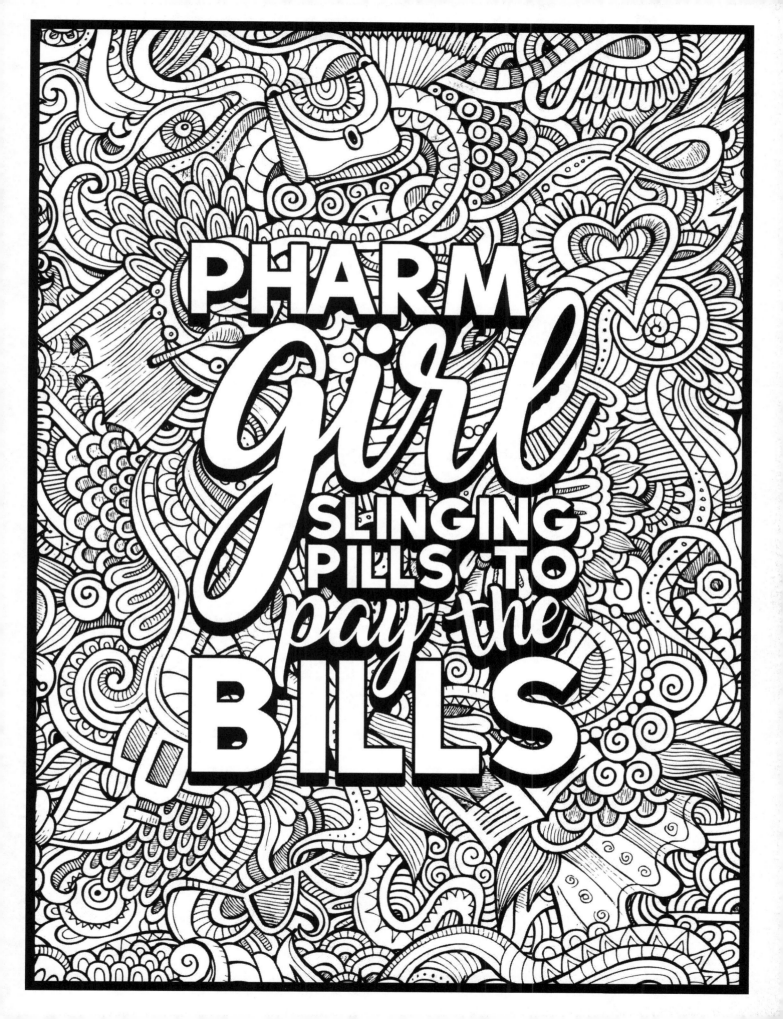

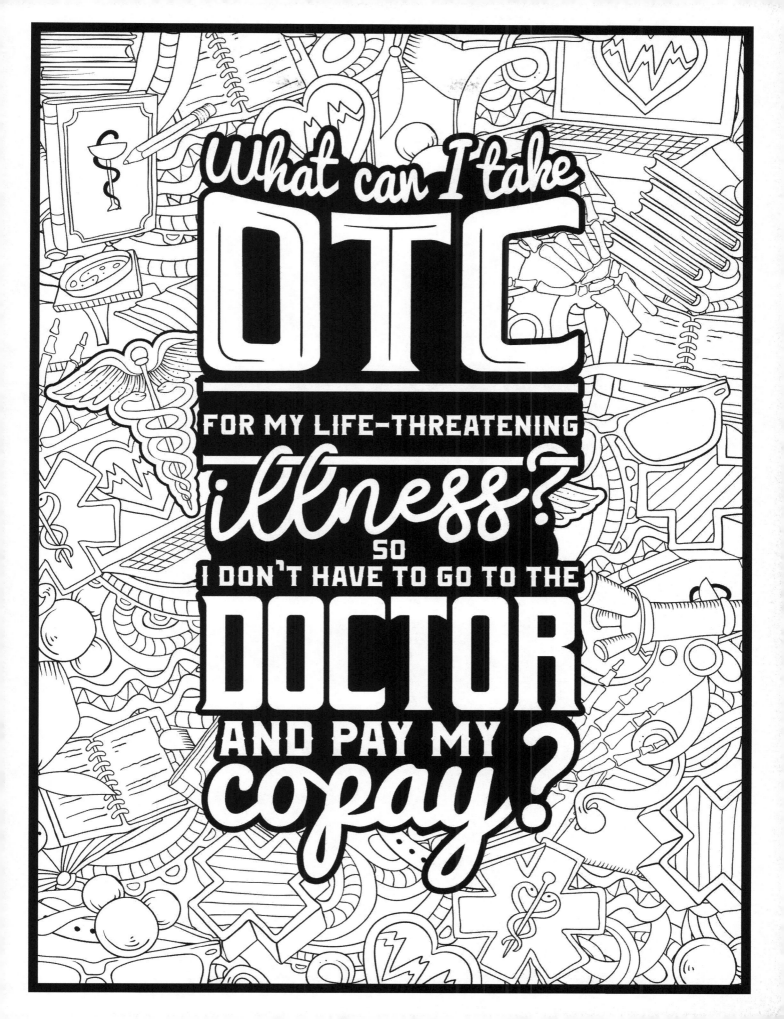

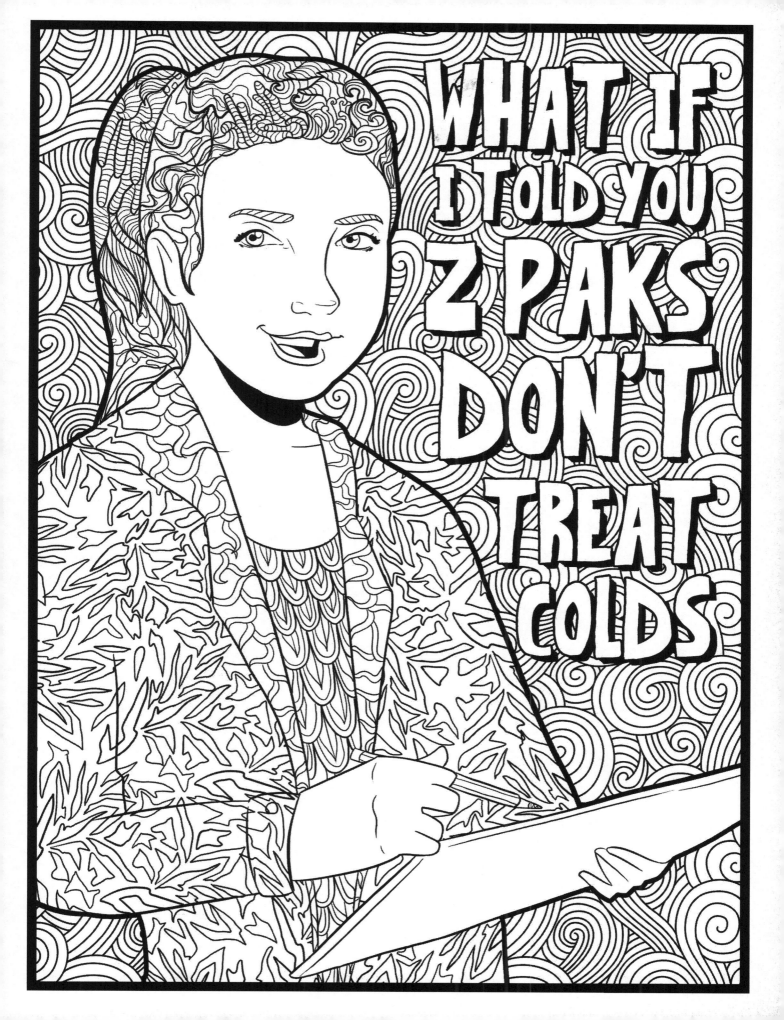

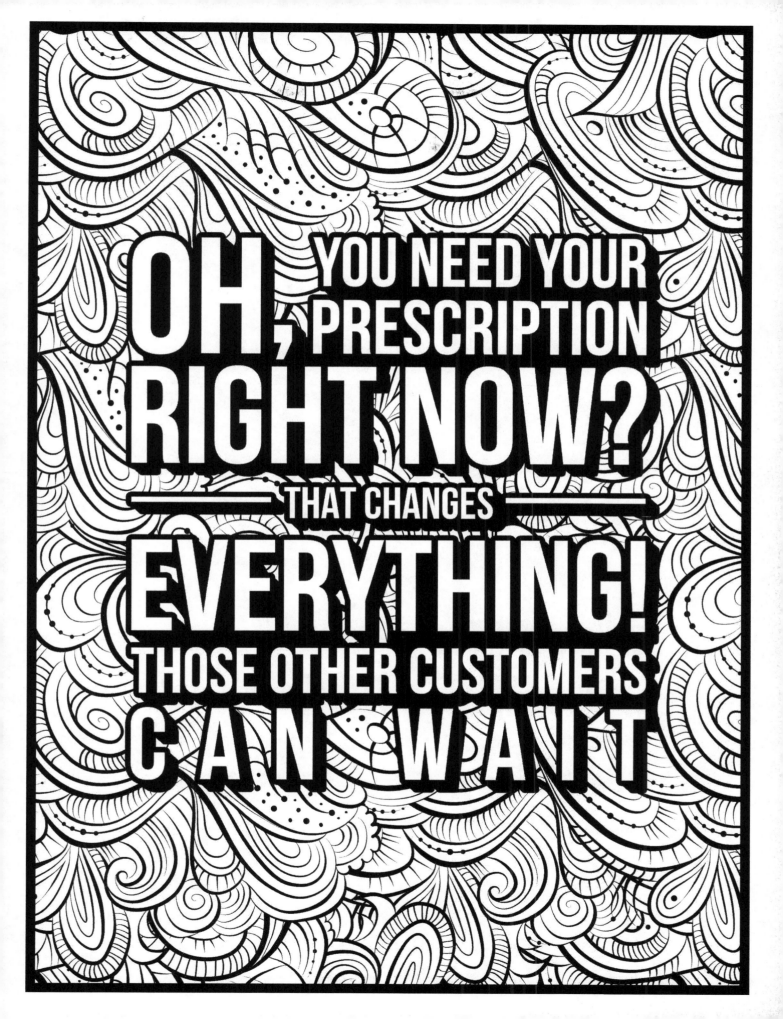

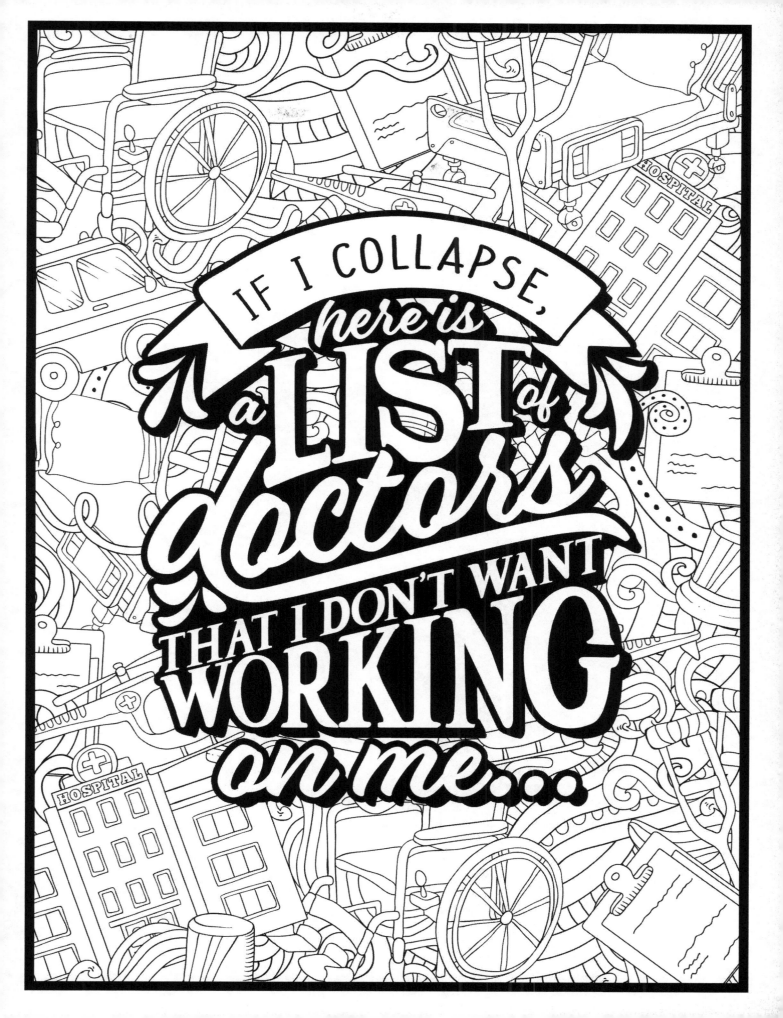

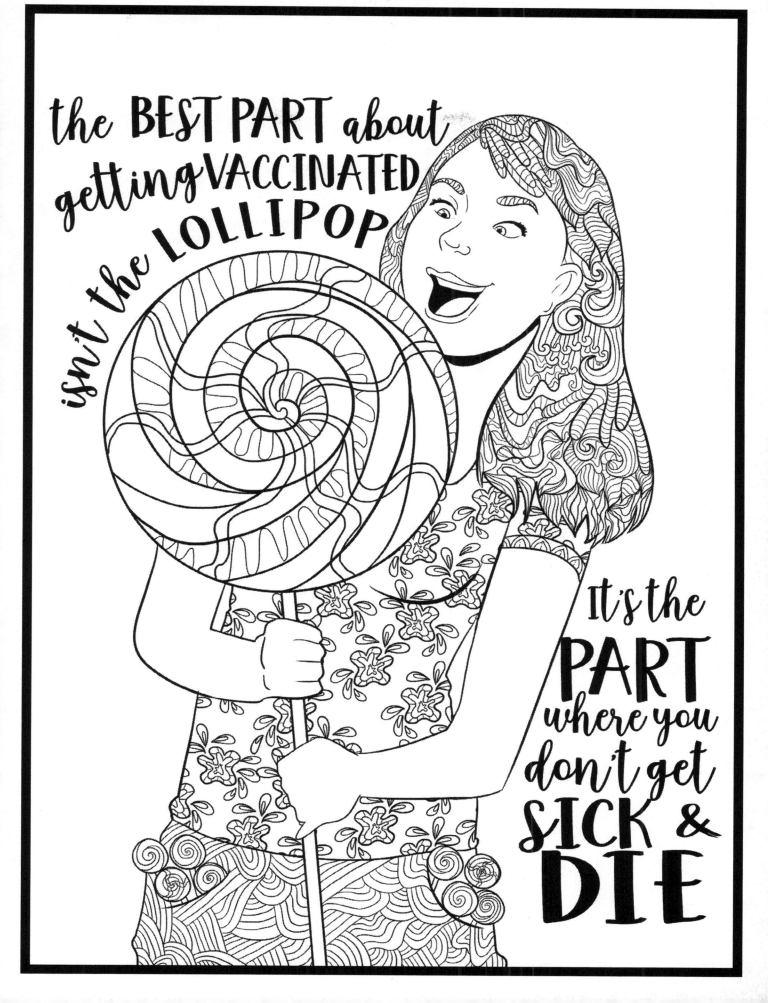

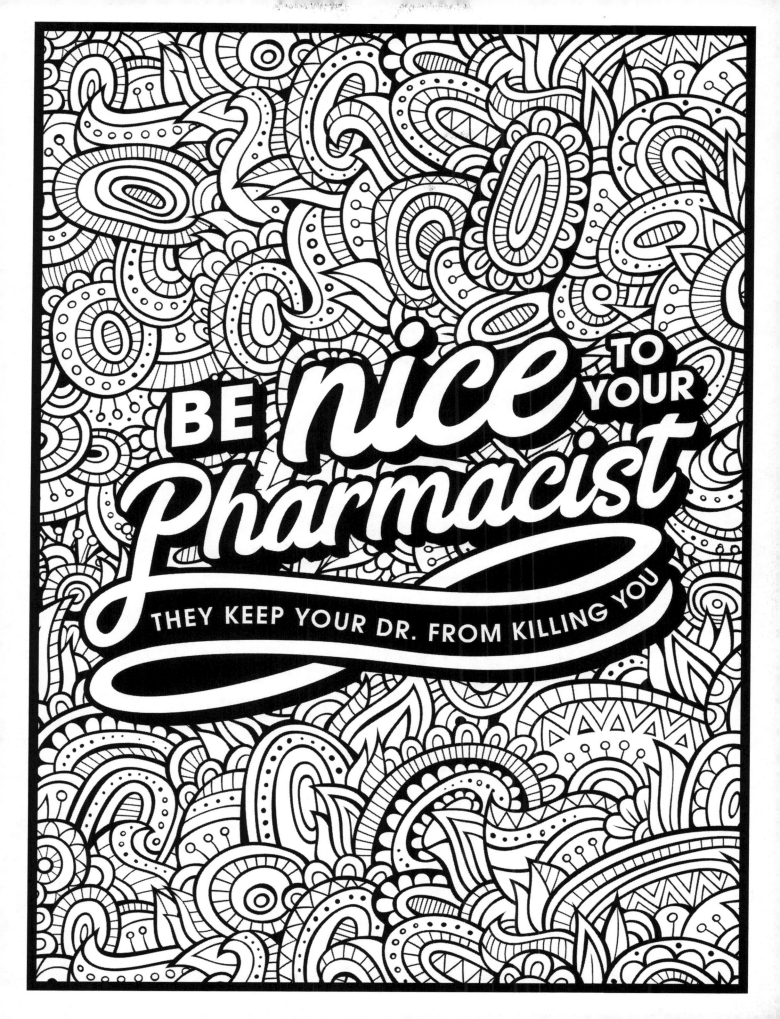

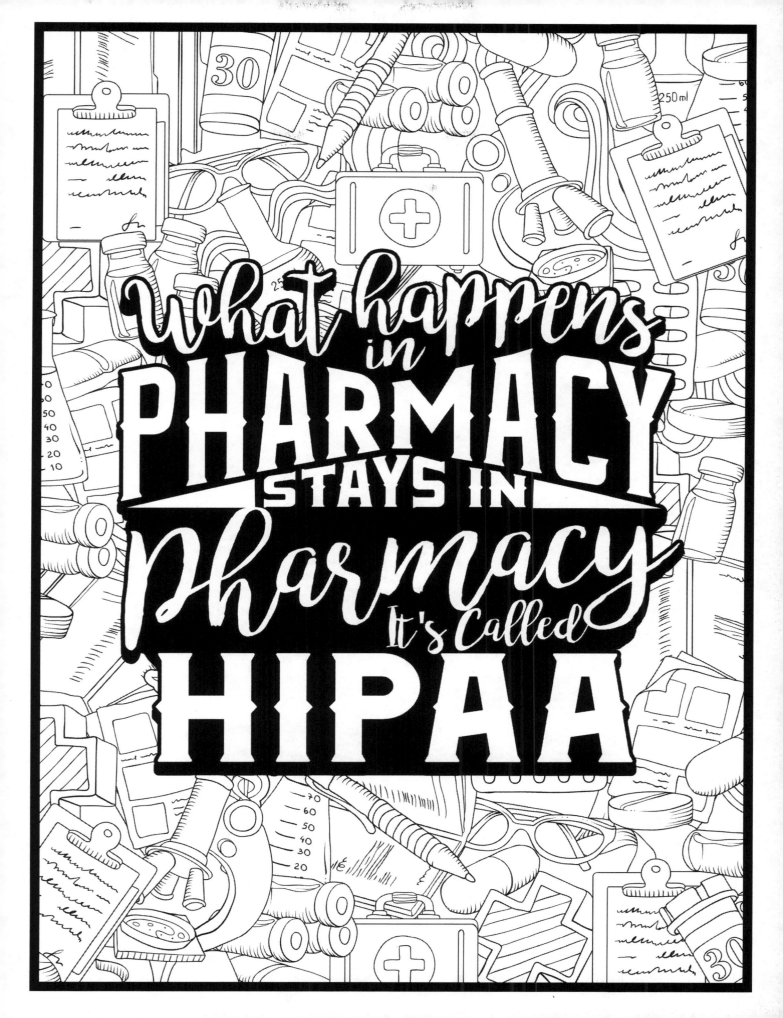

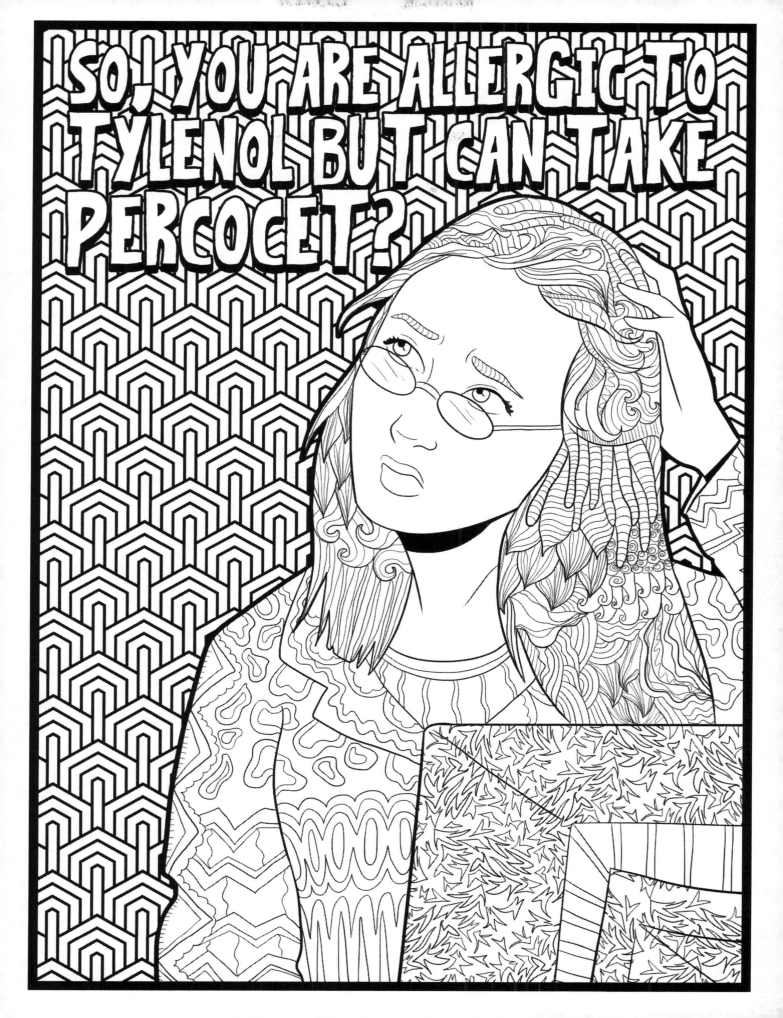

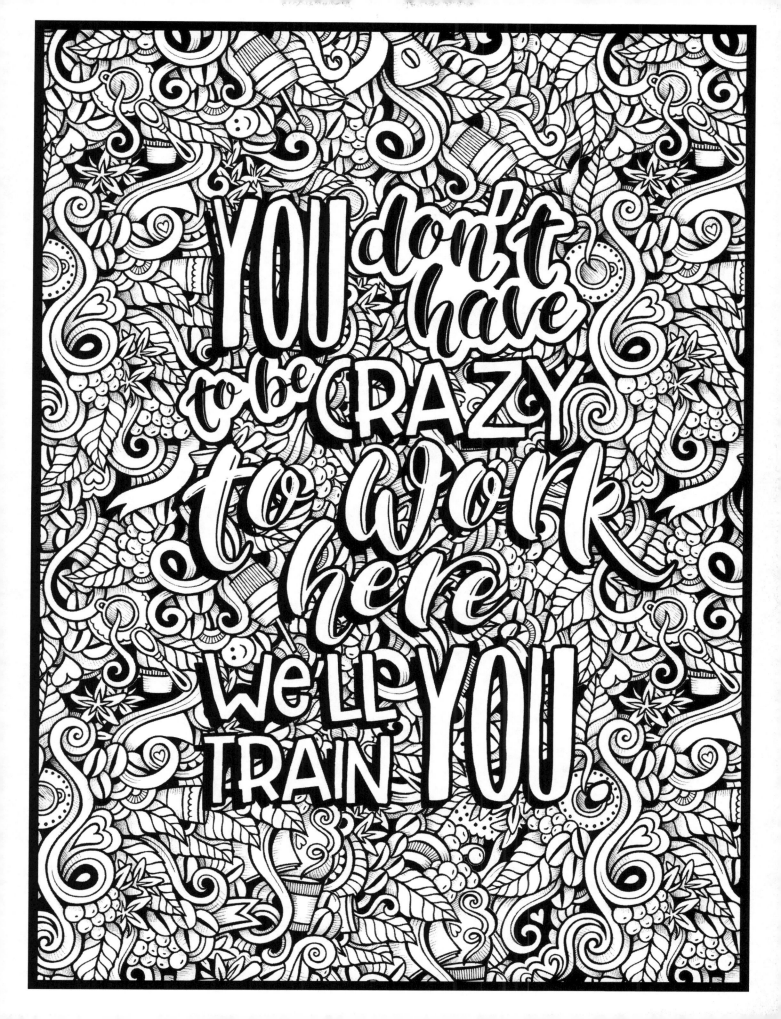

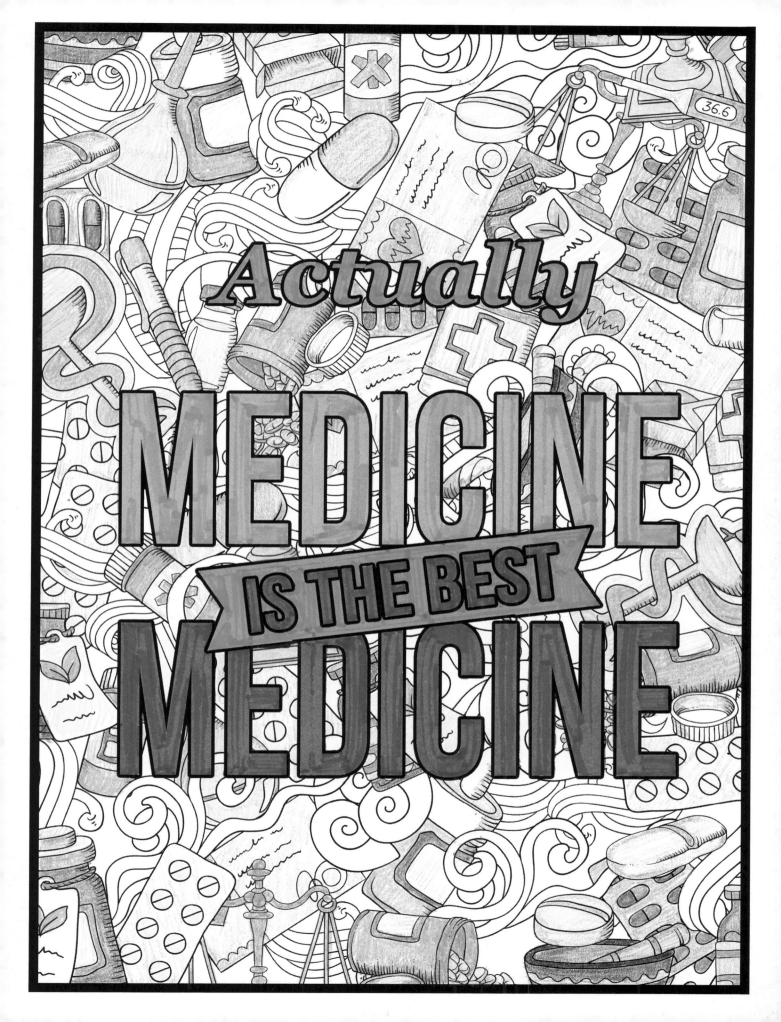

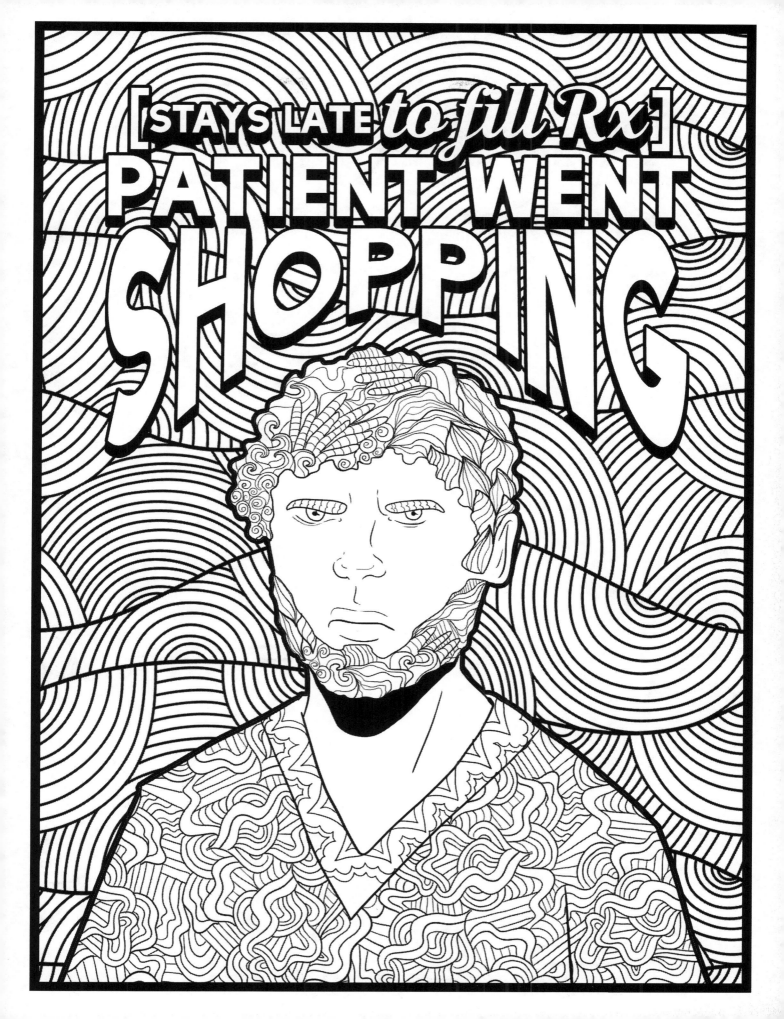

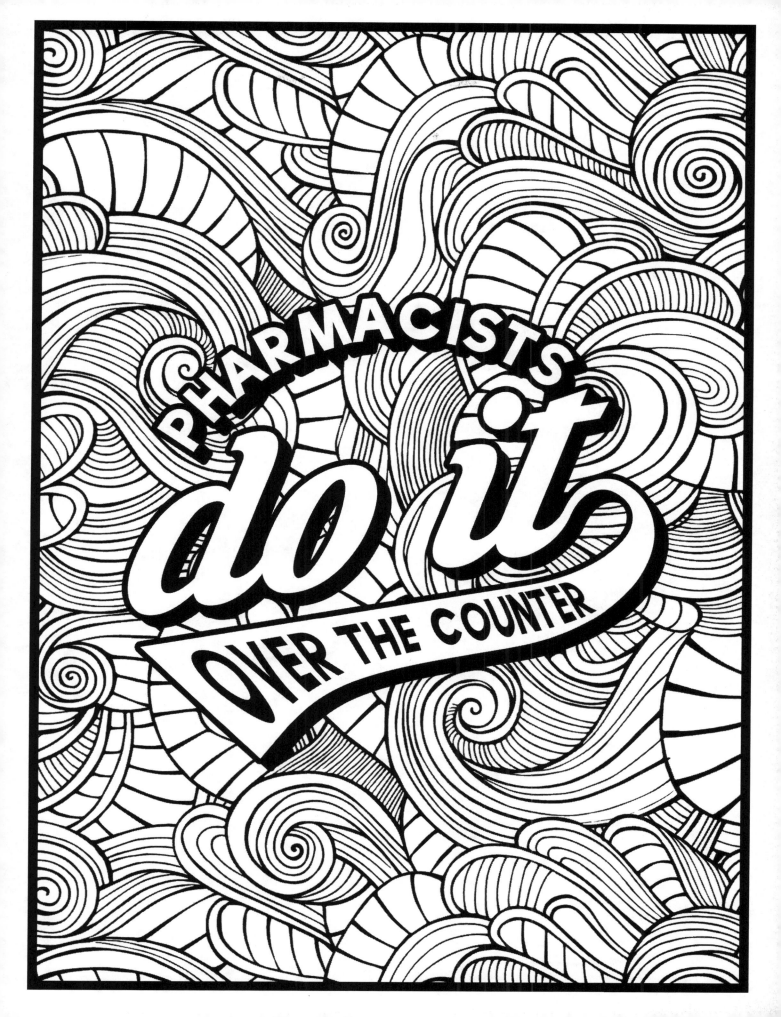

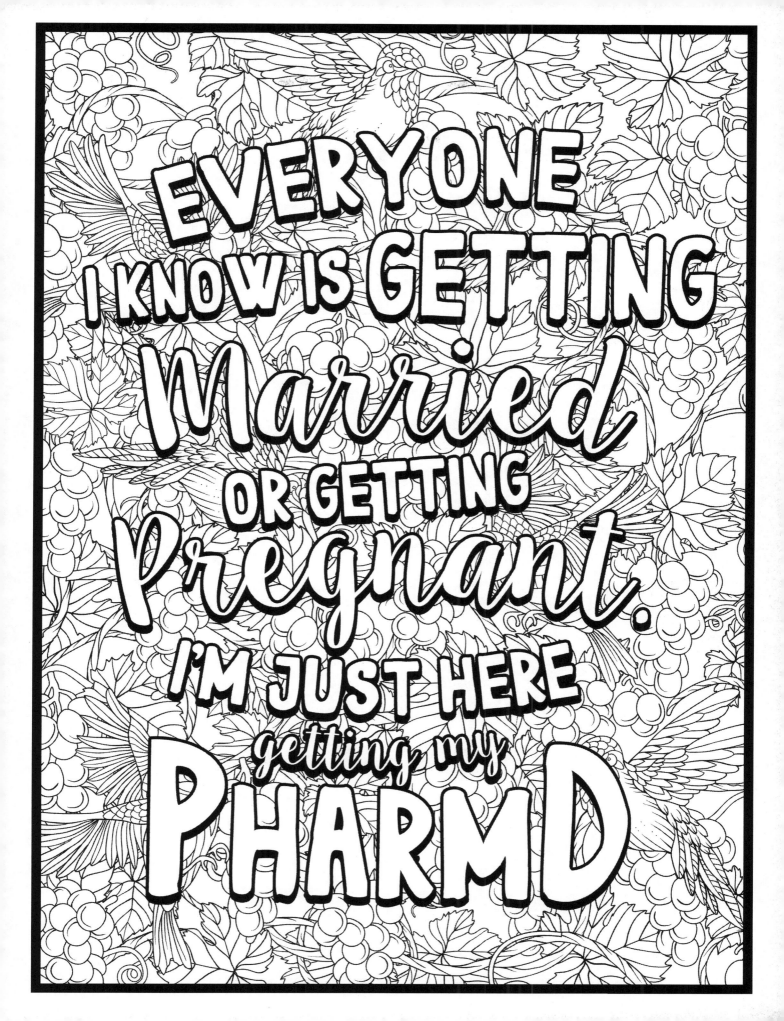

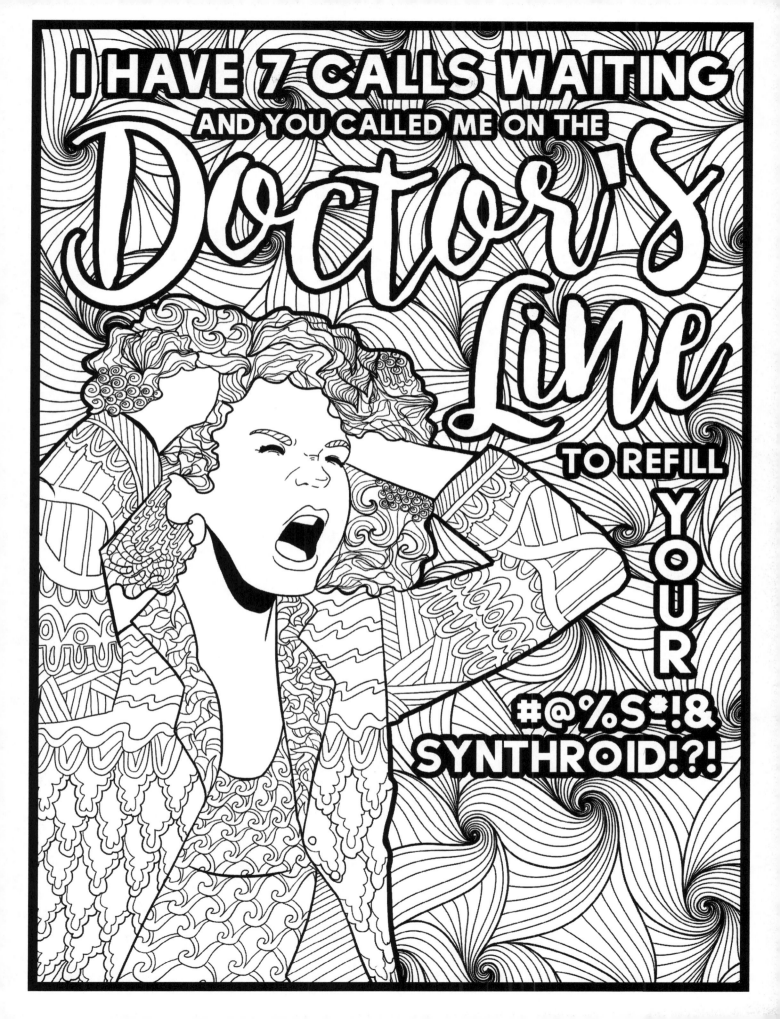

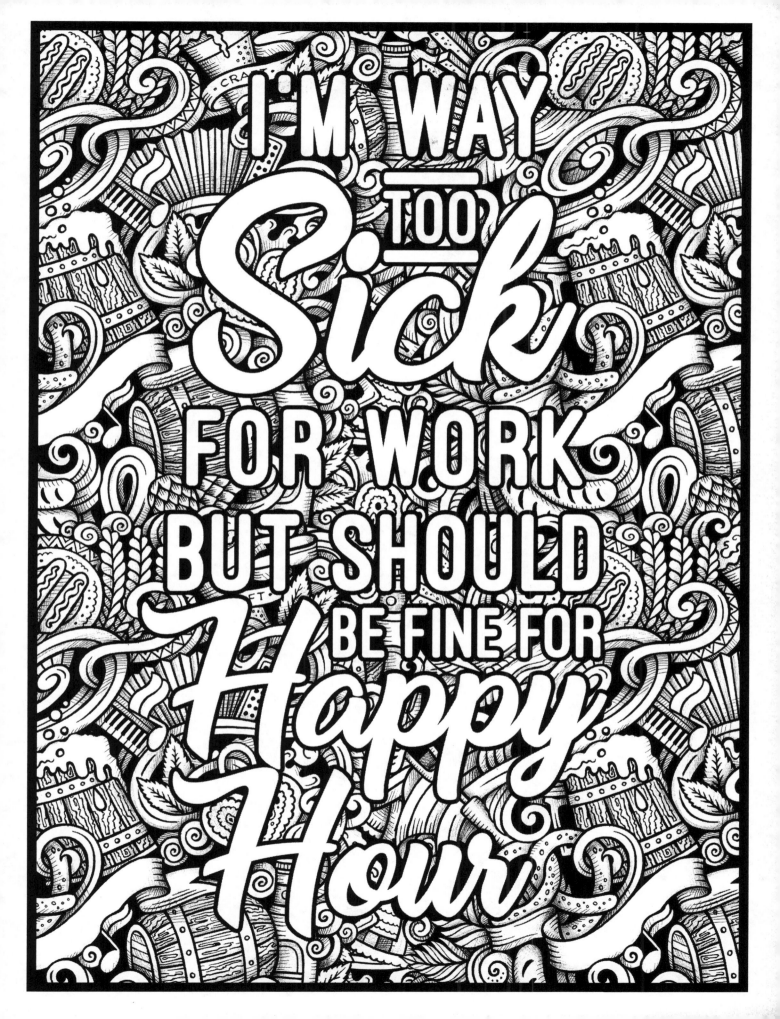

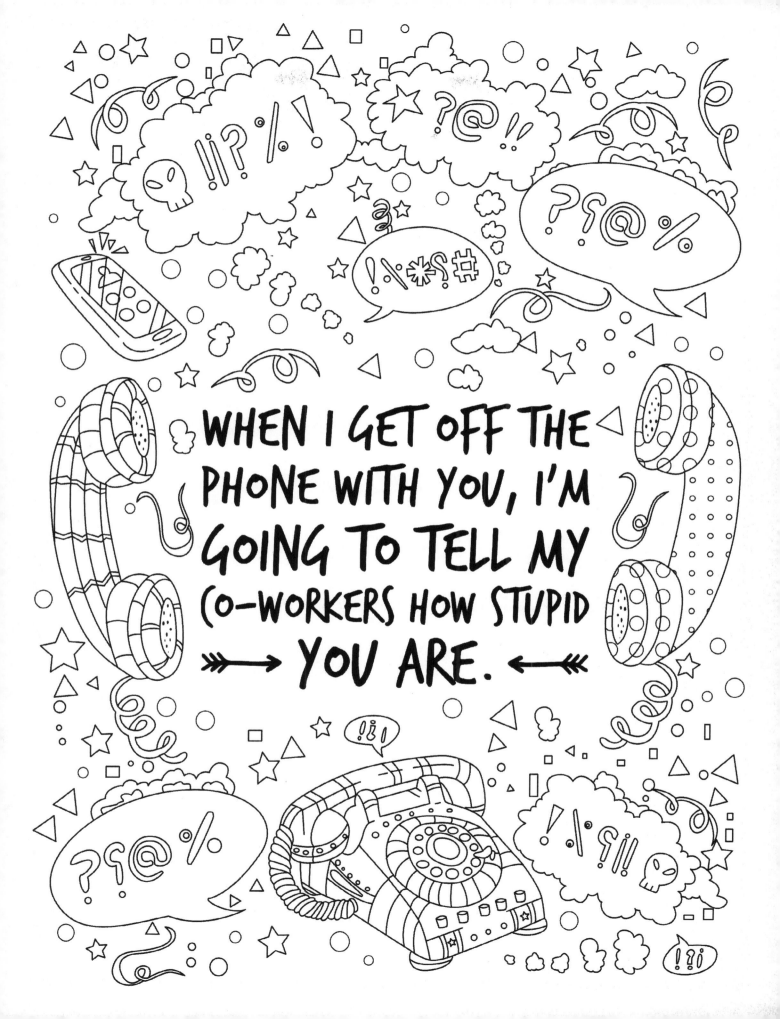

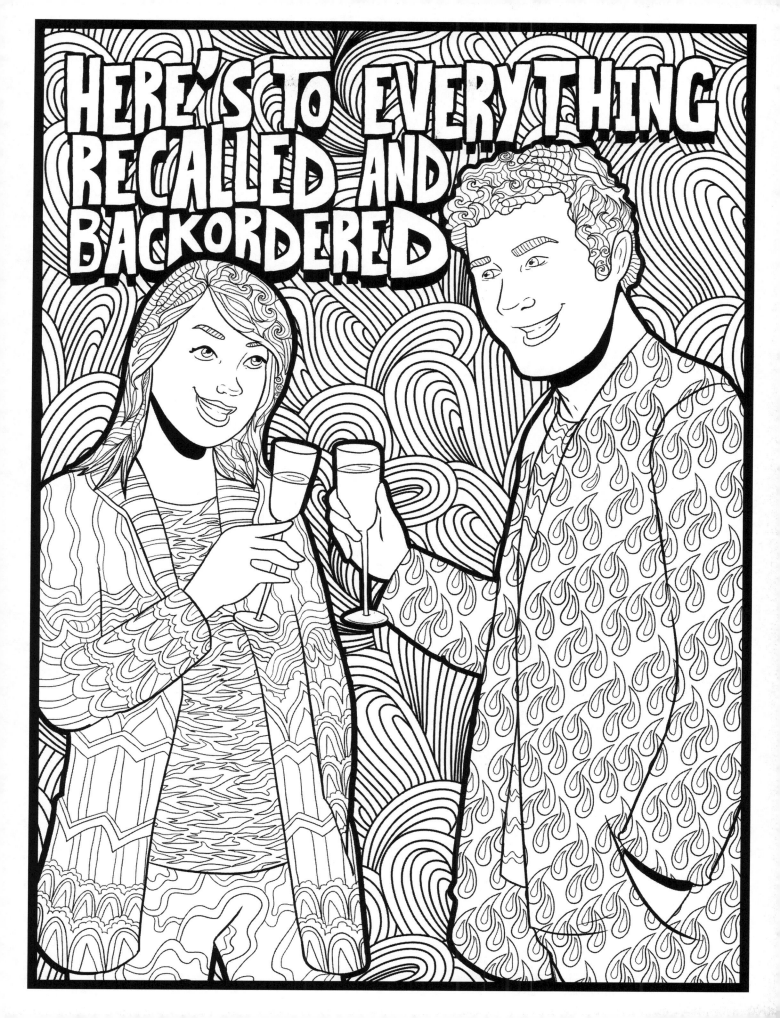

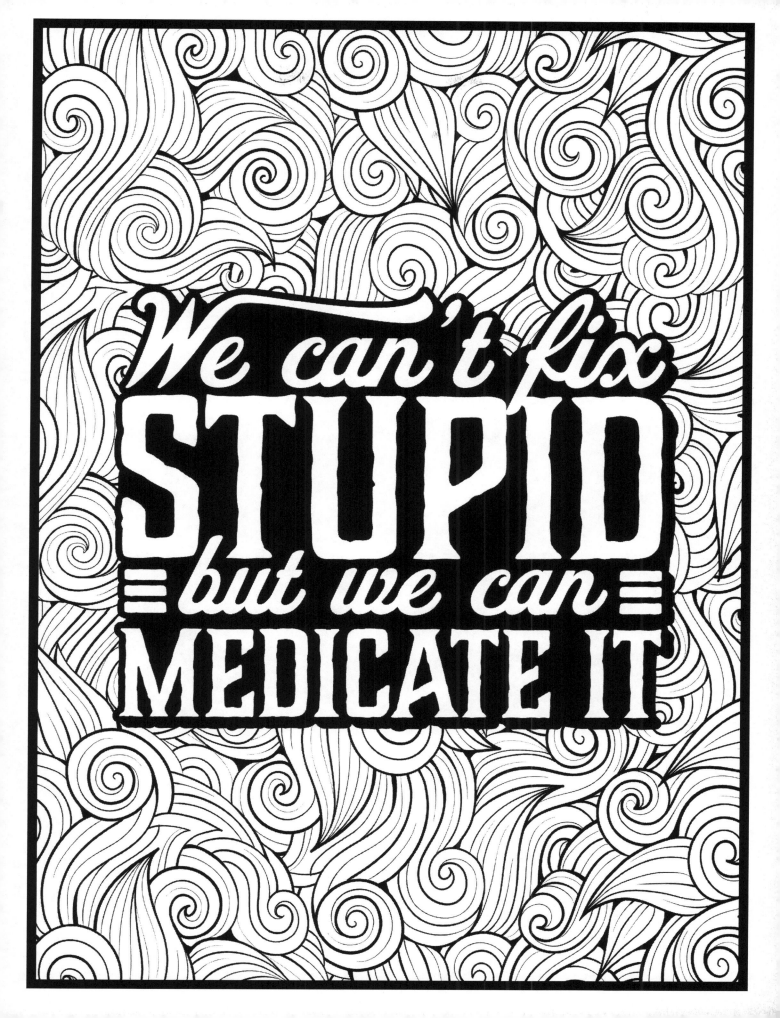

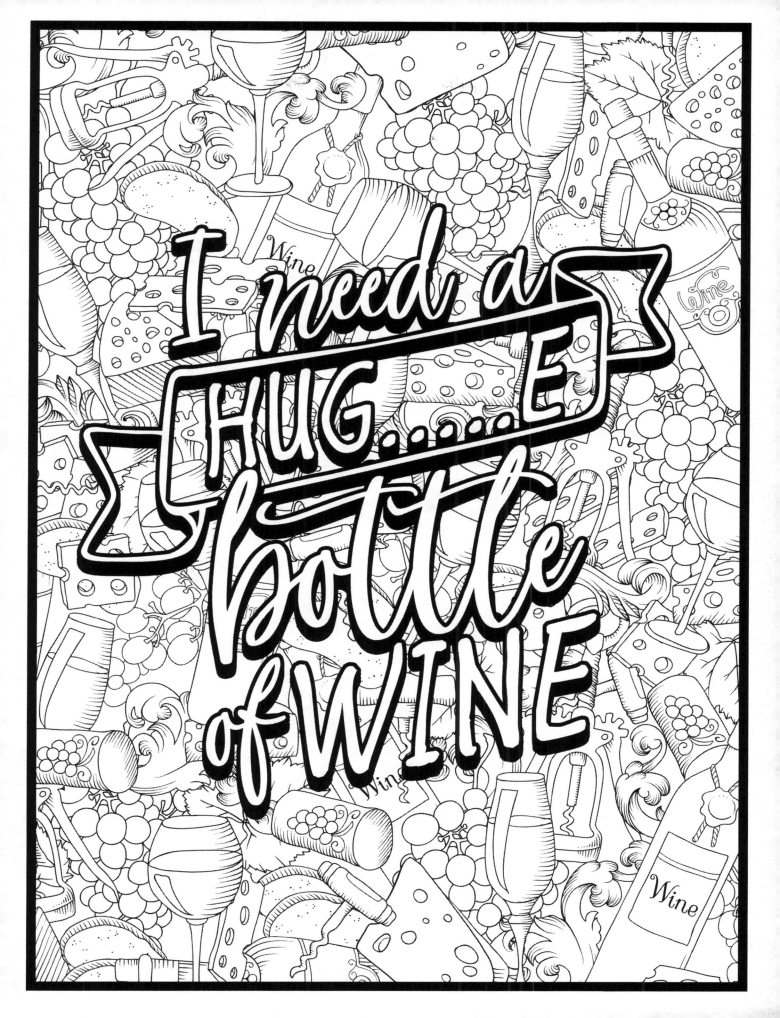

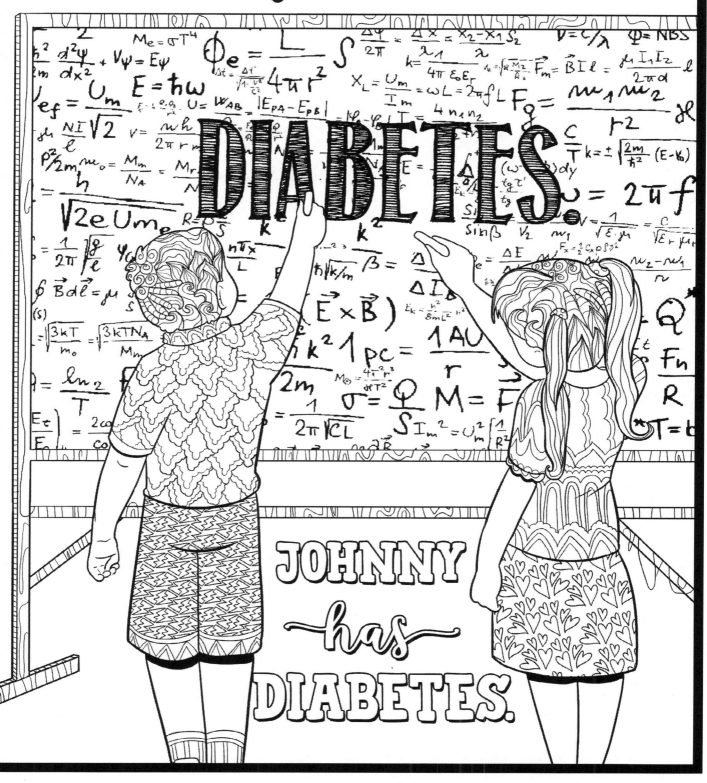

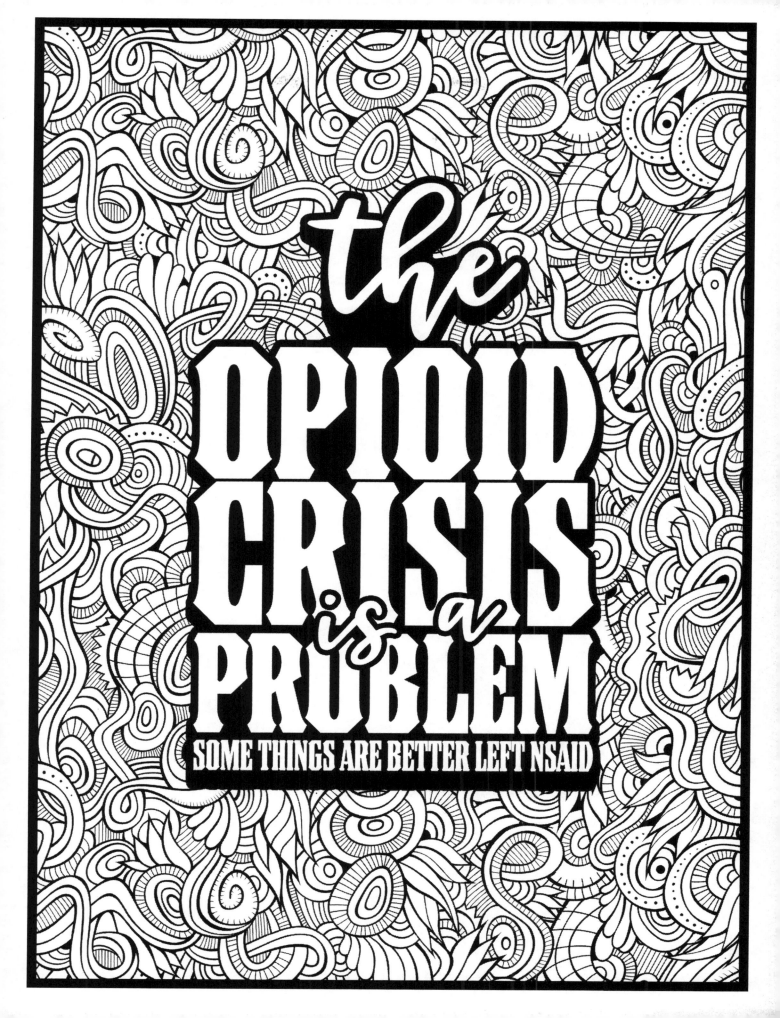

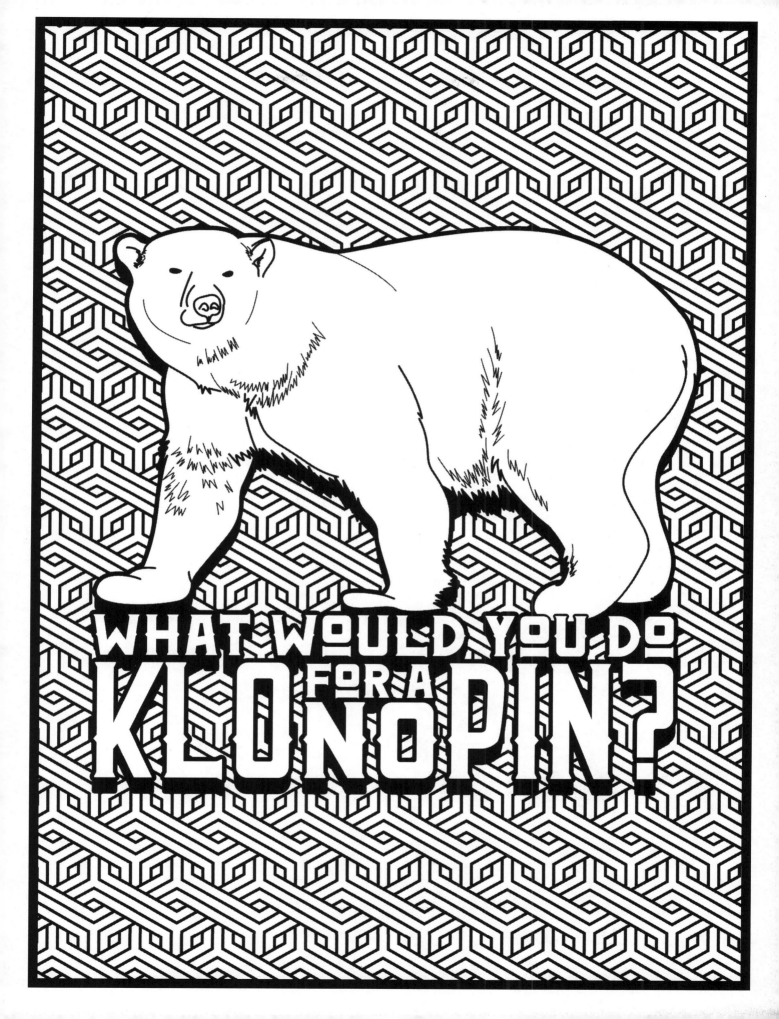

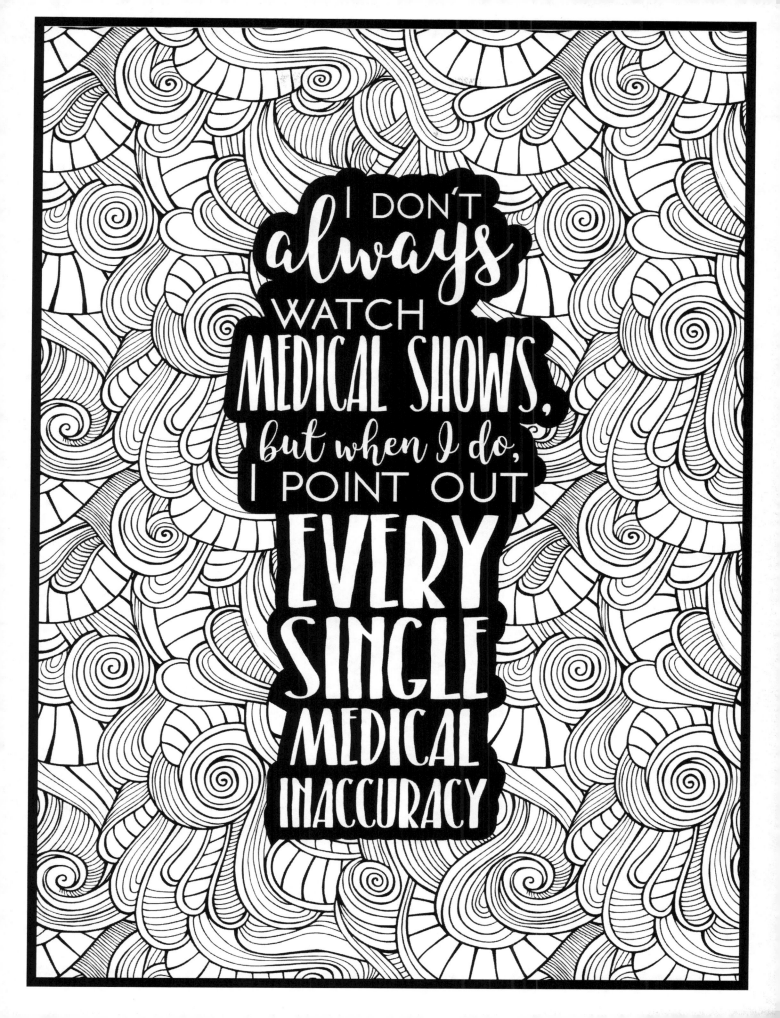

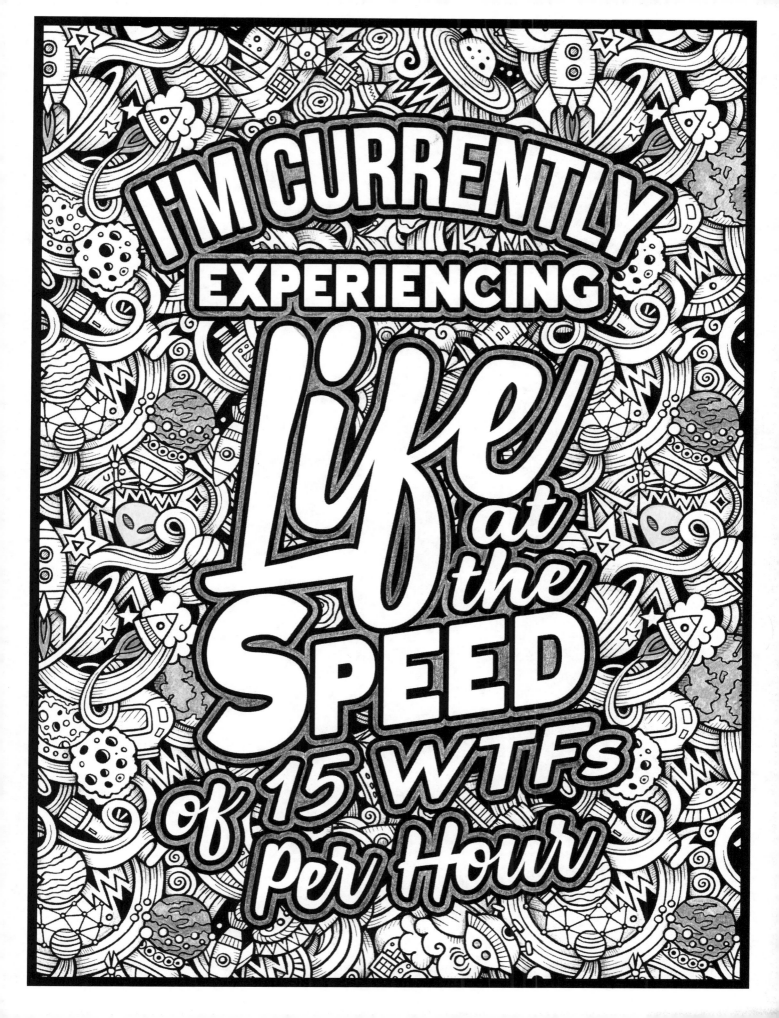

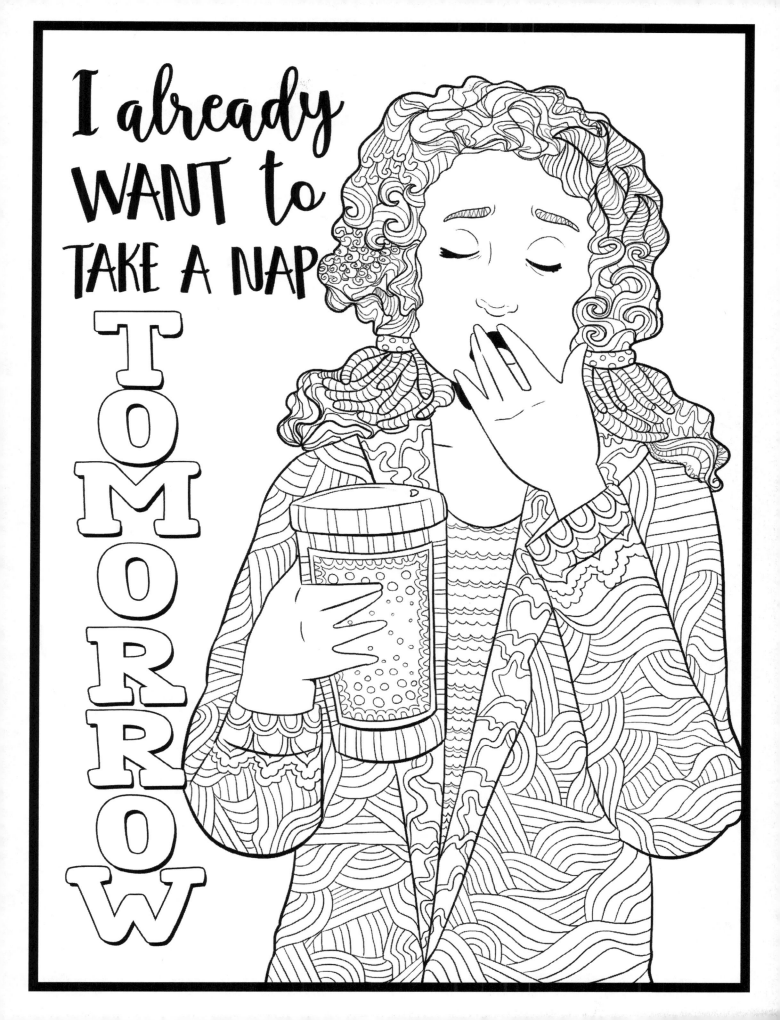

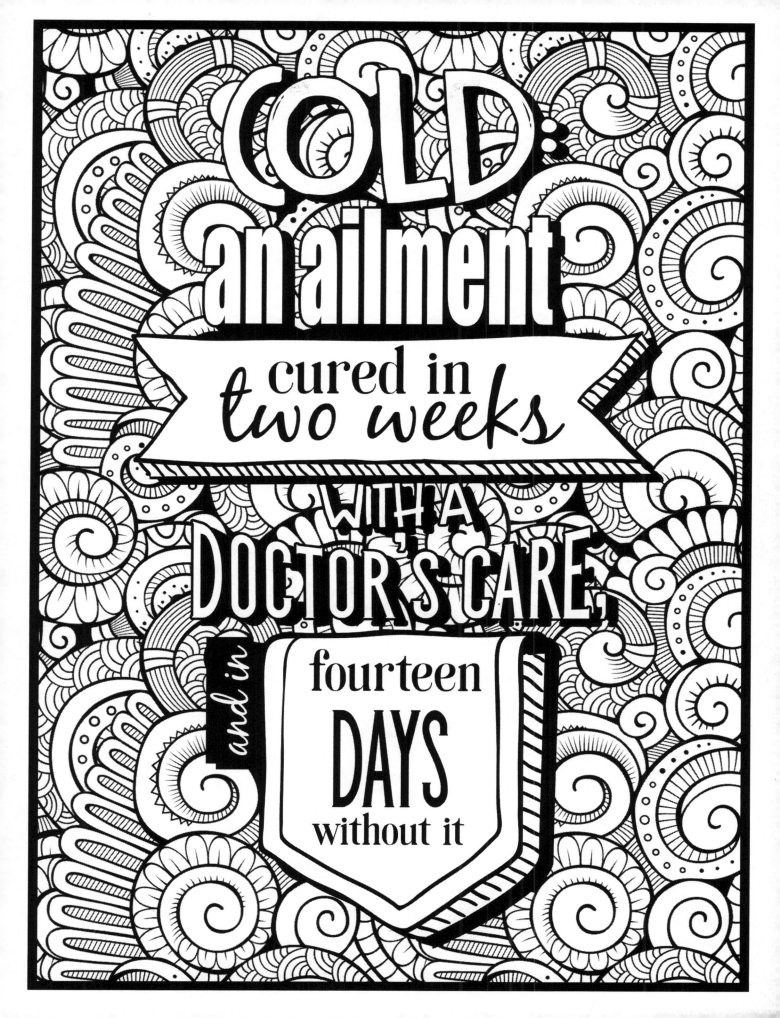

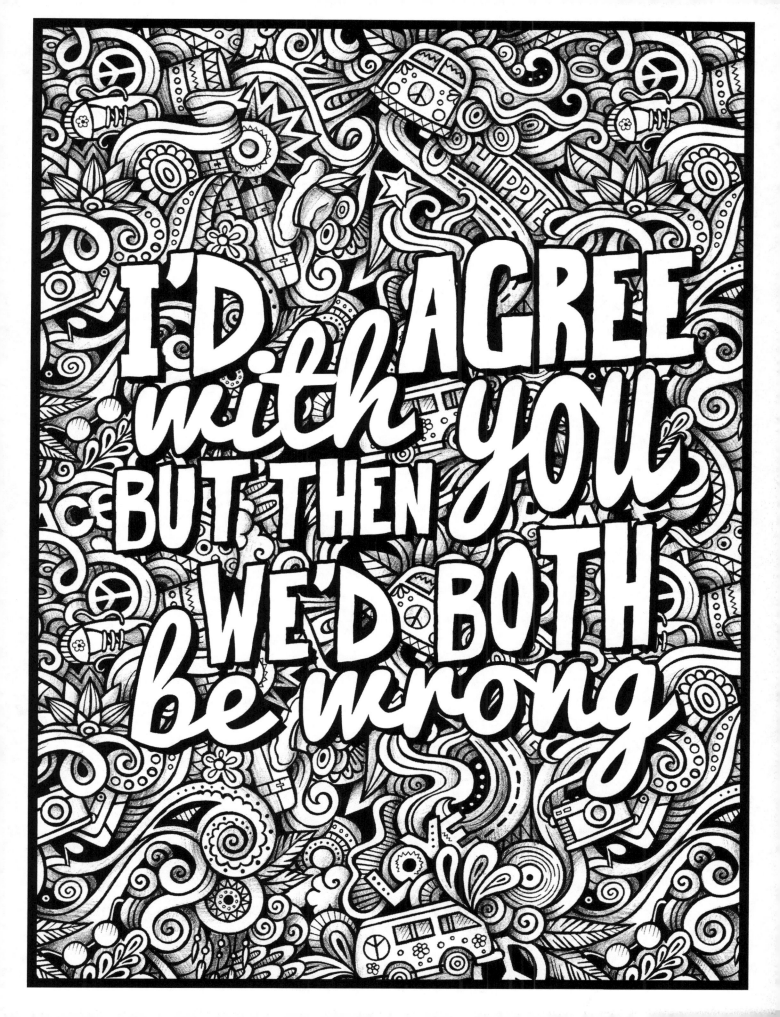

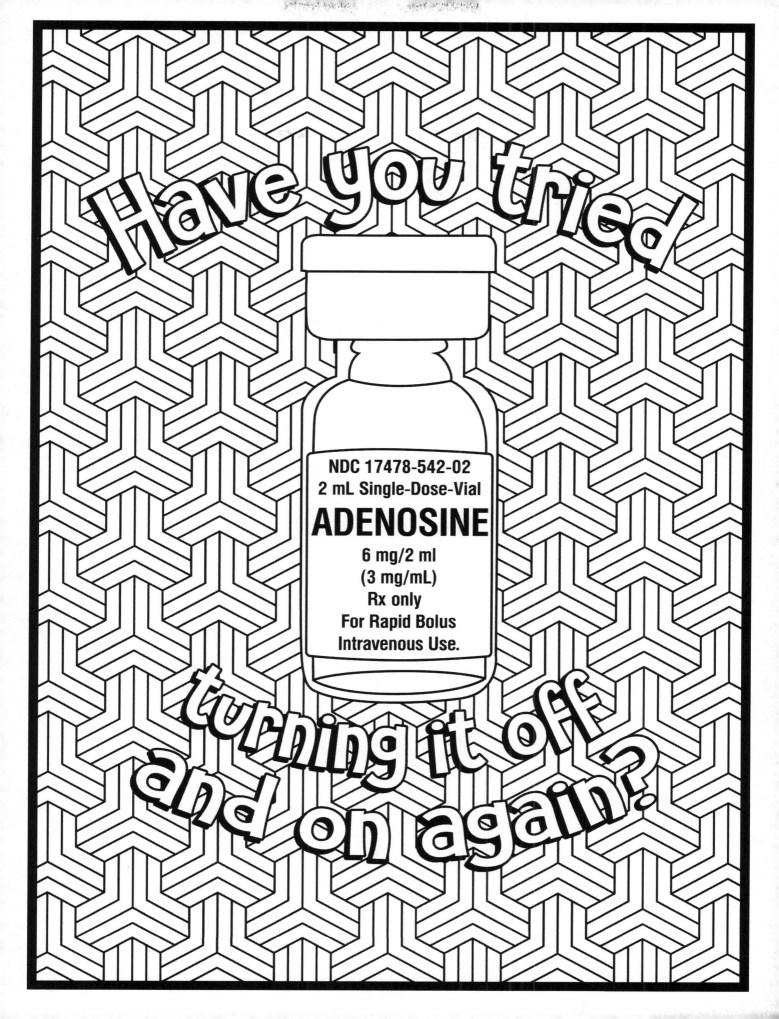

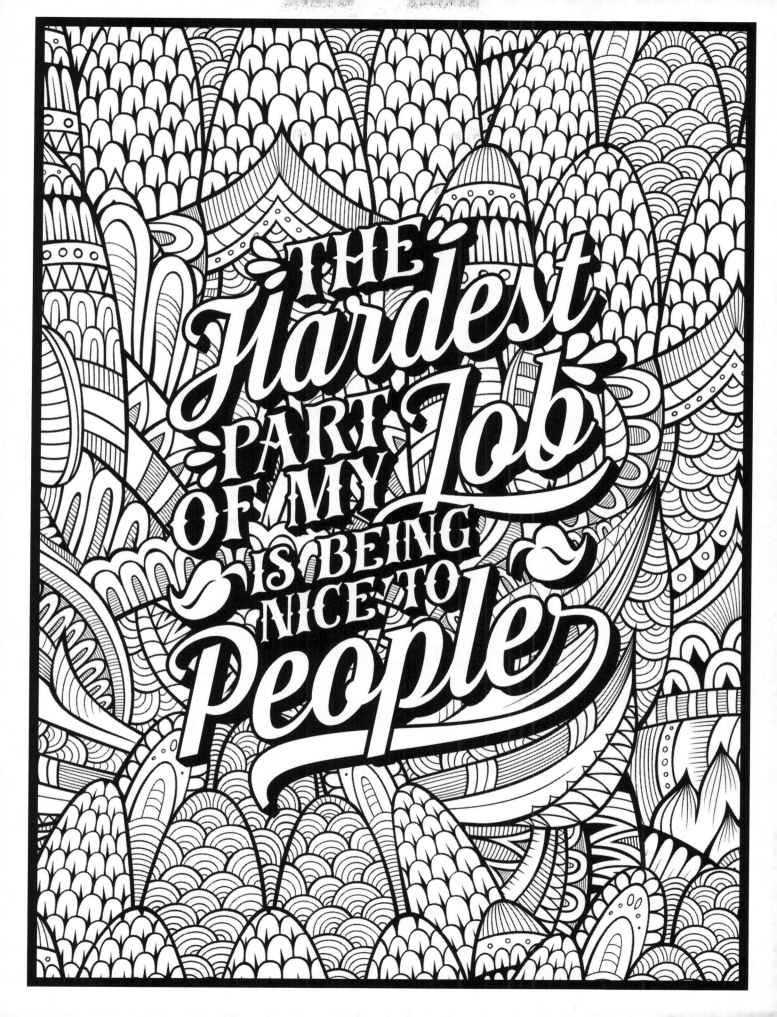

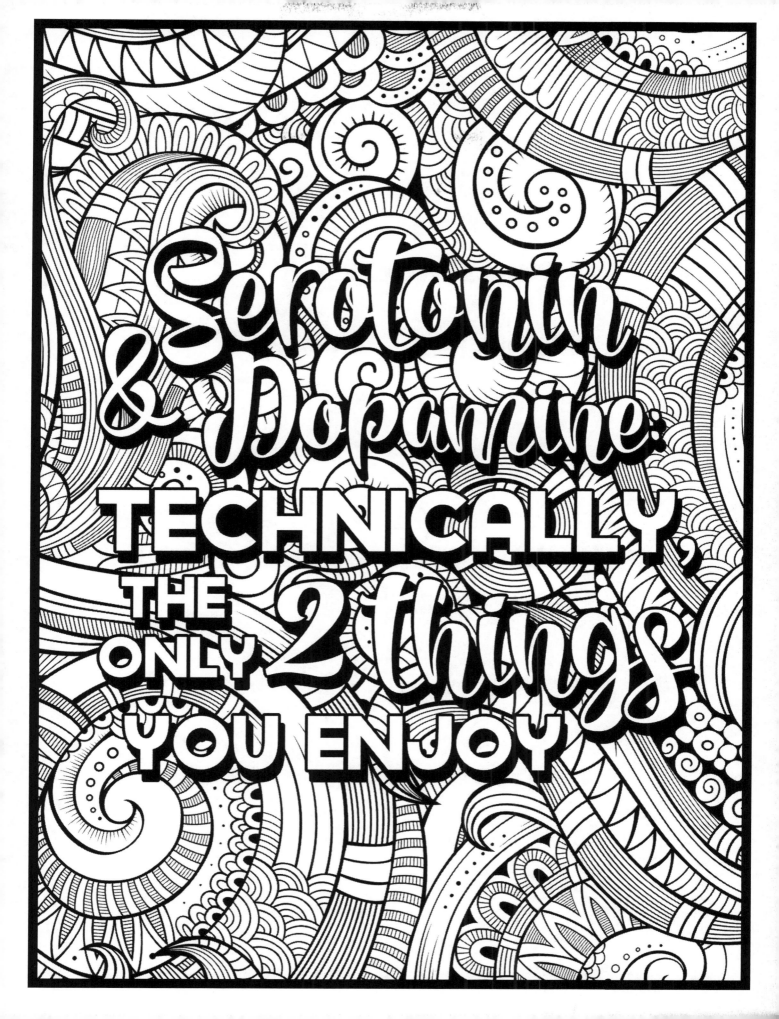

FREE PDF DOWNLOAD
OF THIS BOOK

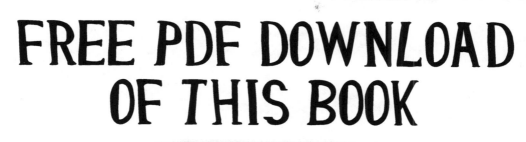

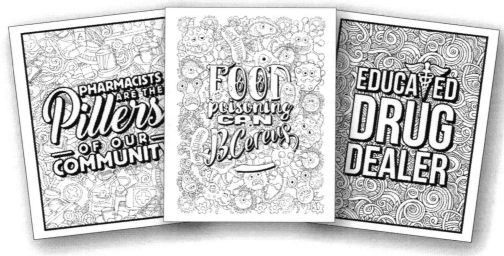

www.pbleu.com/pharmacy

YOUR DOWNLOAD CODE: PHM373

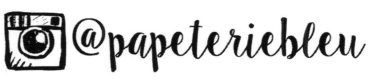 @papeteriebleu

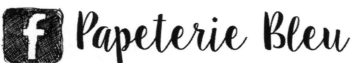 Papeterie Bleu

Want free goodies?
Email us at freebies@pbleu.com

@papeteriebleu

Papeterie Bleu

Shop our other books at
www.pbleu.com

Wholesale distribution through Ingram Content Group
www.ingramcontent.com/publishers/distribution/wholesale

For questions and customer service, email us at
support@pbleu.com

Made in the USA
Columbia, SC
19 April 2022

59193213R00061